Advance Praise for *Feed Your Family Right!*

"It's about time someone wrote a readable healthy lifestyle book for all ages. If you want to know what good health means, you should read this book. If you want to know about healthy eating, you *must* read this book."

—Cathy Nonas, M.S., R.D., C.D.E., director, Diabetes and Obesity Programs, North General Hospital, and assistant clinical professor, Mt. Sinai School of Medicine

"[A] straight-forward resource for parents that brings good nutrition to the family table."

—Roberta L. Duyff, M.S., R.D., C.F.C.S., author of *American Dietetic Association Complete Food and Nutrition Guide*

"The authors make it easy for parents to be the all-important healthy role models they need to be for their children. This is a great book to keep handy and refer to often."

—Keith-Thomas Ayoob, Ed.D., R.D., F.A.D.A., associate professor of pediatrics, Albert Einstein College of Medicine

"*Feed Your Family Right!* is a wonderful, warm, and engaging story about family members of various sizes and their struggles with weight. Elisa Zied gives clear and helpful assistance in feeding families right."

—Sharron Dalton, Ph.D., R.D., author of *Our Overweight Children* and professor of nutrition, food studies, and public health, New York University

"Elisa Zied provides a sound resource that will help you feel secure that you are feeding your family according to the best scientific evidence available."

—Barbara Rolls, Ph.D., author of *The Volumetrics Eating Plan* and professor of nutritional sciences, Pennsylvania State University

"With her keen understanding of family culture, Elisa Zied helps families adopt healthful lifestyle patterns to prevent and control disease."

—Wahida Karmally, P.H., R.D., C.D.E, director of nutrition, the Irving Center for Clinical Research, Columbia University

"A terrific book for the entire family. *Feed Your Family Right!* is a wonderful reference for helping each family member achieve and maintain a healthier body weight. Highly recommended."

—John Foreyt, Ph.D., Baylor College of Medicine

Feed Your Family Right!

How to Make Smart Food and Fitness

Choices for a Healthy Lifestyle

ELISA ZIED, M.S., R.D., C.D.N.

with

RUTH WINTER, M.S.

BICENTENNIAL
1807
WILEY
2007
BICENTENNIAL

John Wiley & Sons, Inc.

Copyright © 2007 by Elisa Zied and Ruth Winter. All rights reserved

Published by John Wiley & Sons, Inc., Hoboken, New Jersey
Published simultaneously in Canada

Wiley Bicentennial Logo: Richard J. Pacifico

Design and composition by Navta Associates, Inc.

No part of this publication may be reproduced, stored in a retrieval system, or trans-mitted in any form or by any means, electronic, mechanical, photocopying, recording, scanning, or otherwise, except as permitted under Section 107 or 108 of the 1976 United States Copyright Act, without either the prior written permission of the Publisher, or authorization through payment of the appropriate per-copy fee to the Copyright Clearance Center, 222 Rosewood Drive, Danvers, MA 01923, (978) 750-8400, fax (978) 646-8600, or on the web at www.copyright.com. Requests to the Publisher for permission should be addressed to the Permissions Department, John Wiley & Sons, Inc., 111 River Street, Hoboken, NJ 07030, (201) 748-6011, fax (201) 748-6008, or online at http://www.wiley.com/go/permissions.

The information contained in this book is not intended to serve as a replacement for professional medical advice. Any use of the information in this book is at the reader's discretion. The author and the publisher specifically disclaim any and all liability arising directly or indirectly from the use or application of any information contained in this book. A health care professional should be consulted regarding your specific situation.

For general information about our other products and services, please contact our Cus-tomer Care Department within the United States at (800) 762-2974, outside the United States at (317) 572-3993 or fax (317) 572-4002.

Wiley also publishes its books in a variety of electronic formats. Some content that appears in print may not be available in electronic books. For more information about Wiley products, visit our web site at www.wiley.com.

Library of Congress Cataloging-in-Publication Data:

Zied, Elisa.
    Feed your family right! : how to make smart food and fitness choices for a healthy lifestyle / Elisa Zied, with Ruth Winter.
        p. cm.
    Includes bibliographical references and index.
    ISBN 978-0-471-77894-3 (pbk.)
    1. Nutrition—Popular works. 2. Health—Popular works. 3. Consumer education.   I. Title.

RA784.Z54 2007
613.2—dc22

2006021035

Printed in the United States of America

10 9 8 7 6 5 4 3 2 1

To my wonderful parents for their wisdom and
unconditional love and support.

Contents

Acknowledgments

I would like to express sincere gratitude to the following people for all their dedication toward making *Feed Your Family Right!* a reality. To Teryn Johnson for believing in this proposal from its inception, and to all the talented people at John Wiley & Sons, including my editor, Christel Winkler, and Tom Miller, Juliet Grames, Lisa Burstiner, and Anne Lesser for creating such a wonderful book. To Stacey Glick, my literary agent, for her constant encouragement and support, and to my collaborator, Ruth Winter, for sharing her wisdom and humor with me throughout the book-writing process.

A special thank-you goes to all the many friends, colleagues, and clients who completed questionnaires or created and/or tested recipes featured in this book. Special thanks also to Maria "Linda" Arevalo, Marlisa Brown, Paolo Casagranda, Elyse Falk, Keri Gans, Zari Ginsburg, Cindy Jennes, Anselma Kuba, Abby Levy, Linda Quinn, Alex Rafal, Anne Sailer, Kyle Shaddix, Maxine Shriber, Barbara Sickmen, Ron Sickmen, Laura Stegmann, and last but not least Claudio Sidoti for creating and testing many of the mouth-watering, family-friendly recipes featured in this book.

To Doris Acosta, Jennifer Starkey, Julia Dombrowski, Irene Perconti, Tom Ryan, and Liz Spittler who make up the fantastic Public Relations Team at the American Dietetic Association, and to my fellow spokespeople who provide me with constant support and encouragement. I am humbled to be involved with such an inspiring, smart, and talented group of nutrition professionals.

I also need to thank two people who are no longer here but who are very much a part of my life. To my late grandmother, Augusta Emansky (Nana), for the many happy returns she sent my way and for the best hugs and tickles a child could ever want (not to mention the best homemade fried chicken and Nana burgers). To my late former professor Richard Schoenwald for inspiring me to always reach for the stars.

To all my wonderful friends for their kindness, support, and love. To my incredible parents, Barbara and Ron Sickmen. To my mother, who raised me to pursue my dreams and who supports me immeasurably as I attempt each day to balance being a wife and mother with having a career. I hope that one day she too will achieve her dream of being a lyricist for Broadway and the big screen. To my father who always questions my dietary advice, to keep me on my toes, and who is always armed with a good joke. And to Maria "Linda" Arevalo for being such a special part of my family.

Last but not least, the biggest thank you in the world goes to my truly amazing husband, Brian, and our two precious sons, Spencer and Eli. Brian has always been so supportive of me and has gone above and beyond to encourage me as I work toward achieving all I set my mind to. No words can express how lucky I feel to have him as my true love, my soul mate, and my best friend. To our older son, Spencer, for amazing me each day with his incredible spirit and kindness. To our younger son, Eli, for his warmth and goodness and for always getting excited when he sees my books in a bookstore. I am truly fortunate to be able to share my life with these three incredible people.

Introduction

When you and your family have a meal, there is more on your plate than just food. This book is written to help you both understand how your past and present family behaviors influence your dietary eating styles today and to show you how each family member can make adjustments in his or her eating and fitness habits to achieve and maintain a healthier weight for life. It will give you more insights into:

- How heredity and genes contribute to your body weight, shape, food preferences, and eating habits
- How family members influence one another's food choices, fitness habits, body image, and attitudes related to nutrition and physical activity, and how family dynamics can support or sabotage a family member's efforts to make healthful choices and enjoy food and eating
- How your age can affect your nutrient and calorie needs, your food choices, your fitness habits, and your overall well-being
- How exposure to cultural pressures such as advertisements, an abundance of highly accessible, highly palatable convenience foods, and hectic schedules affect your family's food choices at the supermarket, at restaurants, and when you grab food on the go

This book is action oriented. It provides you and your family with realistic, achievable, and healthy steps to change your current diet and physical activity habits that sabotage your best efforts and intentions to eat well, live well, and achieve or maintain a healthier body weight. By now, you have undoubtedly read many diet books that focus on helping you lose weight but pay little attention to the fact that you, as an individual, are part of a family, and your family's habits affect your own habits and vice versa. This book gives you a road map to help you and your entire family make changes together, as a unit, with the end goal being a healthier and more fit family.

I needed to write this book for many reasons. I grew up in a house in which mixed messages about nutrition, food, and body weight were paramount. My overweight mother was overly concerned about her weight. She was a compulsive overeater, and a closet eater (she often ate out of view from others), had many fears about food, and seldom enjoyed what she ate. She often expressed guilt when so-called forbidden foods passed her lips. Having a child with a tendency to be chunky (that was me!), my mother felt a need to protect me and to save me from the overweight life she had endured for so long. She always kept an eye on what I ate, seldom brought any kind of junk food into our home (the only snacks I can remember were rice cakes and pretzels), and cooked healthful, fresh meals for our family daily.

As my mother's daughter, I could not help but internalize her weight issues, and to some extent, her issues became my issues. With the exception of when I was ten to twelve years old, I always had a little extra padding growing up, especially when I entered my teen years. And although my mother was always very supportive of me, looking back I realize she may have been too supportive and too wrapped up in my developing weight struggles to help me.

On the flip side, my father, who was a little overweight but basically healthy, always enjoyed his meals and had a voracious appetite. He never really spoke about my extra weight, which perhaps didn't bother him much because he married my mother when she was a little overweight.

My weight had yo-yoed throughout my childhood, but through cutting my food portions, incorporating some exercise, and changing the way I thought about myself and my body and learning to accept myself for who I am and how I look, thighs and all, I have lost 30 pounds and have successfully maintained a healthy body weight for more than ten years. In that decade, I also gave birth to my two sons, and within a year of each pregnancy, I was able to fit back into my jeans!

Fortunately, age, education, and experience have taught me that there's more to a person than a number on a scale. As an undergraduate at the University of Pennsylvania, I studied psychology and took all the nutrition classes offered with the ambition of becoming a psychologist and working with clients who suffered from eating disorders. After graduation, I began my graduate studies in counseling psychology at New York University, as planned. After one semester, I decided to switch to clinical nutrition. I had truly found my calling and knew I would someday become a registered dietitian and help people achieve healthier body weights and overcome their food issues and obstacles. For the last ten years, I have successfully done just that. Through my private nutrition consulting practice, I have been fortunate to work with hundreds of individuals and families to help them make sense of all the nutrition confusion in the media, work through the food and lifestyle challenges they face in their own lives, and improve the way they eat and live. I've also helped them identify and change negative, undermining thoughts and feelings about their own weight and those of their family members to ones that are more positive and that nurture healthy weight behaviors.

As a spokesperson for the American Dietetic Association, I have been given an amazing platform to interpret, translate, and clarify the myriad messages about body weight and weight loss that consumers are bombarded with each day. This book is written to help families cut through the hype. My goal is for parents to find balance in their own food choices, attitudes, and physical activity behaviors and pass that balance on to their kids, so that they, too, can learn to make more sensible, informed choices, feel good about their bodies, and grow into healthy eaters who enjoy food, fitness, and life.

This book will empower you and your family to make subtle but important changes in your eating and physical activities to support a healthier body weight; to understand what is realistic for you in terms of your body weight, shape, and fitness level (taking into account your genes and family history); and to learn how to support one another in maintaining your new, more healthful behaviors, a healthier body weight, and healthier you.

part one

The Journey Begins

1

Family Genes

Who is to blame for your family's weight struggles? The common perception is that if you or your loved ones are overweight, it's because you're lazy and weak willed, and if you simply got up off the couch and pushed yourself away from the dinner table, you'd lose weight and be fit once and for all. There's no doubt that individual food choices and physical activity habits have a great impact on how much you weigh. But our environment makes it more difficult than ever to maintain a healthy body weight and a high level of physical fitness. First, there is the abundance of readily available, highly palatable, heavily advertised high-calorie and high-fat food to entice us. Second, we move our bodies less and less because technology has given us personal data assistants, cell phones, and remote controls so we don't have to get up to change TV channels. Now there are even vacuum cleaners that work without us pushing them.

The Gene-Body Connection

Although eating more and moving less may contribute to many weight woes, that's only part of the story, especially for families in which being overweight or obese is passed down from generation to generation. Jeffrey Friedman, M.D., Ph.D., director of the Laboratory of Molecular

Genetics at Rockefeller University, in his research on why we become overweight, says that genes play as big a role in determining how much we weigh as they do in determining our height. At least 430 genes—the carriers of heredity—that play a part in obesity have been identified by Friedman and other scientists. In fact, an emerging field, nutrigenomics, studies how genes determine our nutritional requirements and how food components interact with our genes and influence our risks for disease and other outcomes.

Genes have been found to play a part in:

- Individual nutrient needs
- Digestion of certain foods
- Susceptibility to diseases
- Susceptibility to eating disorders (such as anorexia)
- Food preferences
- Metabolism
- Response to certain foods and activities
- Desire to eat and stop eating
- Ability to keep weight off once it's lost

Our bodies are shaped by our genes. I am short and pear shaped, just like my mother. When I was a child and young adult, my mom's mother, my mom, and I used to show off how we were three generations and had the same hands and long rock-hard fingernails. Although pretty hands and nails were certainly desirable traits Nana passed on to my mother and me, that's not all that was passed on to us. My mom's dad passed on to my mother and me big thighs, a trait that plagued many of my grandfather's siblings, even the men (you win some, you lose some). As in my family, having a particular body shape, having excess fat where you don't want it, and being overweight are characteristics that many families pass down, generation after generation, because of a combination of genes and environmental factors.

The good news is that having a genetic predisposition to being overweight does not mean that if you are already overweight, you won't or can't lose at least some weight to improve your health. It does not mean your children will inevitably gain unhealthy amounts of weight as they get older. It does mean, however, that it may be more difficult or more challenging for you and your family to achieve and maintain what you consider to be ideal body weights. Both my mother and I battled and subsequently beat the bulge, although we did not, by any means, become model-thin. My mother lost more than 100 pounds by eating smaller portions and becoming more active (she loves water aerobics and other classes). She has kept her weight off for more than twenty-five years. Although she would like to be thinner and have less body fat and a more toned appearance, she understands that her body is comfortable at her current weight. She goes up and down about 5 pounds, eats well, stays as active as she can (she suffers from phlebitis, a blood clotting condition that from time to time limits her mobility), and still has the prettiest nails and hands of anyone I've ever known.

As for me, I currently weigh 115 to 117 pounds—what I considered ideal when I was an overweight fifteen-year-old girl. I have lost a total of about 30 pounds since high school, when I topped off at 145 pounds, and have kept off all the weight for about ten years. I achieved my weight loss simply by reducing my portions, eating more healthful foods like vegetables, and increasing my physical activity—power walking and tap dancing are my favorite pursuits. Although I, too, would like to weigh 5 pounds less just to look better in a bathing suit, I know that I'd have to make too many sacrifices to lose any more weight. That nighttime Oreo cookie? Gone. The small handful of Hershey Kisses midday? No more. And forget about that pat of butter on my bread at my favorite restaurant. So although I'd love to weigh less just to look better for myself (my husband loves me just the way I am, so he says!), I know I am unwilling to make any more dietary cutbacks. I try to always remind myself that I was able to lose weight and keep it off and have two kids in the process simply by reducing portion sizes and adding more fitness into my daily routine. My goal now is to maintain my current weight and build more muscle mass through strength training. And what about my other family members? My brother still struggles with obesity, and my father, who is a few pounds overweight, eats well but tends to go overboard on portions, and he seems content to go up and down losing and gaining the same 5 or 10 pounds.

Fortunately, you and your family can do a lot each day to improve your eating and fitness habits and reap many benefits in terms of your overall health, body weight, and appearance. This chapter will help you take a close look at your personal and family histories as well as family patterns that relate to body weight. It will show you that even though you belong to the same family, each member has a varied genetic makeup and will respond in a unique way to any changes made in food choices or fitness habits. With help from this book, you and your family will learn how to set realistic food- and fitness-related goals and create personalized lifelong eating and fitness patterns.

Take Paul, for instance, a thirty-four-year-old father of two small girls, ages four and two. He has two overweight parents. Paul's maternal grandparents both lived well into their nineties, despite the fact that his grandmother was overweight and had type 2 diabetes most of her adult life. Paul's mom, in her sixties, is apple shaped (see the box "Apples versus Pears" on page 15) and has been about 20 pounds overweight since her thirties, after having two children. Even though she takes medication to control her blood pressure and cholesterol levels, she puts salt on everything she eats and clears her plate at every meal. She also does little physical activity. Early in life, Paul's paternal grandfather was diagnosed with type 2 diabetes that eventually caused him to become blind. He died of a heart attack in his late seventies. Paul's dad, now in his early seventies, also developed type 2 diabetes as an adult. When he was initially diagnosed more than a decade ago, he lost some weight but subsequently gained most of it back. He's about 20 pounds overweight and takes medication twice daily to control his blood sugar. Like his wife, he clears his plate, avoids sugar like the plague, and is inactive except for some walking.

Is Paul doomed to follow in his family's genetic footsteps? No, because he is aware of his family history and is determined to change his weight and his ways. His weight was 162 pounds on his five foot eight frame just after college, when he worked 100 hours a week, ate mostly takeout, and did very little physical activity. Over the next few years, he took up running and his weight leveled off in the low 150s. He ran three marathons, and during his training his weight dipped to 152 pounds. Over the last six years or so, since he and his wife had two girls, his physical activity has diminished considerably. His weight hit the upper 150s, and after several borderline high cholesterol readings, and given his family history of diabetes and high blood pressure, he decided to be proactive and make some changes. He kept a food record for three days (see page 22) and also filled out a physical activity form (see page 28). He makes sure to choose oatmeal or whole-grain cereal with low-fat milk and fruit for breakfast instead of his usual bagel with cream cheese. Rather than snacking mid-morning on sugary foods like breakfast bars, he usually has low-fat yogurt and nuts. He eats what he likes but limits animal foods with a lot of saturated fat like red meat and cheese. He goes to the gym four or five mornings per week, where he runs and lifts weights. He has maintained his weight at approximately 150 pounds for about two years. At a recent physical, his internist complimented him on his good physical condition.

What about the Influence of Family Culture?

Marie was a busy young mother with three small children. Although she had always been overweight, she gained even more weight with each successive pregnancy. Her mother, father, and sisters and brothers—there were a lot of them—were all obese. Growing up in a home in which it was expected that all family members would clean their plates, which was not so hard to do because the food their mother cooked was fatty and delicious, no doubt contributed to Marie and her siblings subsequently becoming overweight. As an adult, Marie became a cook just like her mother, and she felt like a failure if her husband and children didn't clean their plates after she slaved, however willingly, over a hot stove. Marie put so much effort into food shopping and meal preparation, not to mention juggling three kids' schedules, that she had little time to exercise. The only real physical activity she got was chasing after her children.

Marie seemed destined to continue to balloon in weight until we worked together. First, we identified her family's genetic and emotional history as well as their cultural tastes. We documented her current eating patterns (see sample food record on page 22) and uncovered situations that prompted her to overeat. She discovered that she would turn to food in response to visual cues such as TV ads and/or aromatic triggers such as the smell of cinnamon muffins at the mall. We discussed her daily schedule for both weekdays and weekends and determined which times of the day were the toughest for her. For example, she often skipped breakfast during the hectic morning frenzy with her kids, and she constantly grazed on food while preparing dinner for her family. We also listed what she perceived to be obstacles that prevented her from preparing more nutritious meals, limiting portion sizes, and increasing daily physical activity.

We came up with several simple solutions that she then incorporated into her life—she woke up twenty minutes earlier than she usually did to prepare breakfast for her kids and herself, and she snacked on cut-up vegetables with a low-fat yogurt dip or hummus while making dinner. We also discussed how important it was for her pro-mote healthful patterns such as eating until you're comfortable and not pressuring her children and husband to finish everything on their plates. She has slowly but surely realized that even if her family does not eat all the food on their plates, it does not mean they don't enjoy the food she makes or that they love her less. Marie has also learned how to take a few minutes to stop and identify how she feels before she eats, and to eat because she's hungry, not because she feels bored, tired, happy, or upset, or because she sees tempting food.

Even though Marie will likely never be slim—she inherited a stocky, muscular build from her mother—she has lost 40 pounds, and has a pleasing, full figure. She takes pride in her looks, has more energy, and is healthy. She feels empowered to make more mindful decisions about food, nutrition, and physical activity, and she has a positive influence on her family.

How Much Do Lifestyle and Environment Combat Genetic Tendencies?

Amy's entire family—mother, father, and two sisters—were all thin. Amy had also been thin most of her life until she began pursuing a high-powered career in the financial industry. She got little sleep because she had to wake up at five each morning to check overseas markets on her computer. She always skipped breakfast. For lunch, she either went out to fancy restaurants with clients or ordered takeout and dined at her desk. She also mindlessly snacked all day on candy from other people's desks and from her own desk drawer. She worked long hours and never found time to exercise. Adding to her caloric intake, she would stop at a local bar after work to socialize and have a few drinks and many peanuts to unwind from the stress of the day.

First, I encouraged Amy to keep a three-day record of how she spent her time. Taking an objective look at how much time she spent on all her daily activities was a real wake-up call for Amy. We came up with some realistic, sensible steps she could take to increase her physical activity. She also kept a food record (see page 22) to give her a glimpse of her eating habits (she skipped breakfast often), what she was over-doing (candy at her colleagues' desks), and where she was falling short in terms of food groups. Amy now prepares a quick breakfast, and she brings nuts or some high-fiber cereal and a low-fat yogurt packed on ice to have as a mid-morning snack at her desk. Instead of taking the elevator to her fifth-floor office, she takes the stairs. She gets up from her desk to talk to colleagues instead of communicating via e-mail. She also takes two or three ten- or fifteen-minute walk breaks at work. And three days a week, she packs a healthy desktop lunch that includes lean protein such as turkey, chicken breast, or tuna, grains such as whole-wheat crackers or multigrain bread, fresh fruit or cut-up vegetables with a low-fat yogurt dip, and skim milk or low-fat cheese. She even keeps preportioned snacks in her desk drawer—nuts, seeds, whole-grain crackers, and tubes of peanut butter. When she dines out with clients, she skips the bread and the drinks. She finds many of her dining companions are happy to do the same because they had felt obligated to join in the routine bread and drink even though they too were watching their caloric intake. Amy always orders some kind of vegetable or salad for an appetizer and eats half of her fish, lean beef, or chicken entrée.

Now, instead of spending time at the bar after work, Amy unwinds at a health club. She has found that socializing at the club is just as rewarding as it had been at the bar. Amy lost 25 pounds in six months. Her coworkers think it is just because she gave up eating their candy and don't realize the other changes Amy has made to achieve her weight loss.

So for Paul, Marie, and Amy, it was possible to make relatively small changes to get on the road to healthy eating and a healthy lifestyle despite their genetics and their past and present family food and activity habits. Like them, you too will learn how to create and maintain a weight management plan for yourself and your entire family that takes into account each family member's unique food and activity preferences and overall lifestyle.

A Reality Check for Your Family

Before you and your family make any changes at all in your eating or fitness habits, take a look at your entire family and where each of you is starting from in terms of your own body weight, shape, and size, and medical history. This will give you some insight about the impact of your genetic family history and what's realistic for you and family members in terms of your own body weight and shape goals.

You can use several simple tools to assess and evaluate your current body weight and shape that will help you set your weight-related goals (see chapter 2): body mass index and measurements including waist circumference and frame size.

Body Mass Index and Frame Size

To see how your weight measures up, you can determine your body mass index (BMI) in appendix B and record your BMI on the form in appendix A. BMI measures your weight in relation to your height and is a reliable indicator for determining how much body fat you have. But even though BMI is useful, it is not foolproof. It may overestimate body fat in those who are very muscular and it may underestimate body fat levels in older people who lose muscle mass with age.

In addition to BMI, knowing where excess body fat is located on the body also provides a window for potential health risks. If you carry fat mainly around your waist, you are more likely to develop health problems than if you carry fat mainly in your hips and thighs. This is true even if your BMI falls within the normal range.

Take Out Your Tape Measure

Another tool you can use is an old-fashioned tape measure. With it, you can easily measure your waist circumference. This is useful for both adults and children. The wider the waist (the more fat you have around your middle), the higher the risk for many diet-related ills including cardiovascular disease, high blood pressure, type 2 diabetes, and other obesity-related conditions. See the box "Apples versus Pears" on page 15 to see what shape you are.

To measure your waist circumference, place a tape measure around your bare abdomen just above the hip bone. Be sure the tape is snug but does not compress the skin and is parallel to the floor. Relax and exhale, and then measure the waist (record this measurement in inches in the chart in appendix A). If you would feel more comfortable, ask your doctor or another health professional to help you take this measurement. Women with a waist measurement of more than 35 inches or men with a waist measurement of more than 40 inches may have a higher disease risk than people with smaller waist measurements because of where their fat is located.

Using a tape measure periodically to keep track of your waist size is a great way to determine how you're doing in terms of body fat level and body fat distribution. Even in young children and adolescents,

Apples versus Pears: What Shape Are You?

Did you know that not all body fat is created equal? Even if, like me, you're plagued with hips and thighs you wish were smaller—your body is pear shaped (it's smaller on top and bigger on the bottom)—that extra bit of padding may actually be a blessing in disguise and is associated with reduced health risks compared with those with an apple shape. Recent studies suggest that excess hip and thigh fat may actually protect against cardiovascular disease and death, as well as metabolic syndrome. Why the benefits? One theory is the fat that accumulates in the lower body may act as a reservoir for harmful fats that would otherwise accumulate in the body. Or perhaps it could be that those who are genetically pear shaped are less likely to gain extra fat around their middles than those who are genetically shaped like an apple.

Having an apple shape (you have relatively thin arms and legs and when you gain weight, it tends to go straight to your gut) increases your risks for several diet-related diseases including heart disease, diabetes, hypertension, and metabolic syndrome as well as breathing problems, disability, some cancers, and a higher death rate. That's because belly fat, also known as visceral fat, surrounds internal organs and secretes powerful chemicals that can increase the risks for disease. The more belly fat, the greater the health risks. Many women tend to have a pear shape (but may develop more of an apple shape when they experience menopause), whereas men tend to be more apple shaped.

No matter what shape you are, you can improve your overall health by staying active and engaging in regular exercise such as walking or cycling, as well as weight training, making better food choices, and achieving and maintaining a healthier body weight.

Sources: B. H. Goodpaster et al., "Obesity, Regional Body Fat Distribution, and the Metabolic Syndrome in Older Men and Women," Archive of Internal Medicine 165, no. 7 (2005): 777–83; "Are you an Apple or a Pear?" myDNA News, reviewed by Rick Nauert Ph.D., American College of Cardiology, September 16, 2005.

research suggests that increased upper body fat is associated with higher levels of blood fat, triglycerides, and lower high-density lipoprotein (HDL), the good cholesterol. Although there are no set standards that establish safe or healthy norms for waist circumference measurements in children, your pediatrician can certainly measure your child's waist at yearly check-ups to see how it changes over time, and compare the measurements with values observed in children by researchers and published in the *Journal of Pediatrics* in 2004. If your child's waist circumference (measured at the end of the lowest most rib at the end of a normal expiration) falls above the ninetieth percentile for age and gender (see the table below), they are at significant risk for obesity-related diseases and conditions.

Frame Size: The Bones Your Ancestors Gave You

A tape measure can also help you determine your genetic bone structure and frame size. If you naturally have a larger frame—if you're big boned like Marie's entire family, including her parents and grandparents

Waist Circumference at the Ninetieth Percentile (in centimeters)		
Age	Boys	Girls
2	50.8	52.2
3	54.2	55.3
4	57.6	58.3
5	61.0	61.4
6	64.4	64.4
7	67.8	67.5
8	71.2	70.5
9	74.6	73.6
10	78.0	76.6
11	81.4	79.7
12	84.8	82.7
13	88.2	85.8
14	91.6	88.8
15	95.0	91.9
16	98.4	94.9
17	101.8	98.0
18	105.2	101.0

Source: Adapted with permission from J.R. Fernandez et al., "Waist circumference percentiles in nationally representative samples of African-American, European-American, and Mexican-American children and adolescents," Journal of Pediatrics 145 (2004): 439–44.

who emigrated from the same town in Italy—it's likely that you cannot weigh the same as a person with a smaller bone structure who is the same height as you. Knowing your frame size can help you and your family members set realistic weight-related goals (see chapter 2). Helping your children measure their frame size is a great way to teach them that we all come in different sizes and no matter what size we are, we can certainly take action to make our bodies stronger and more fit. To determine your frame size, see appendix C and record it on the chart in appendix A. Frame size measurements apply only to adults, though you can help your children measure their own wrists to show them how bone sizes vary from person to person, even within the same family.

Whether you have a small, medium, or large frame depends on bone structure and density. Men and women differ in frame size and people of the same gender may also differ. Genes determine about 40 to 80 percent of bone length and structure according to Stefan Judex, Ph.D., a researcher in the Department of Biomedical Research at the State University of New York at Stony Brook. The remaining fraction—20 to 60 percent—is determined by environmental factors including diet and exercise.

Although you can't do much to change the actual shape of your body, you can change the appearance of your body, muscle, and skin. Overweight or not, making simple dietary changes and increasing the frequency and types of physical activity in which you and your family engage can result in tremendous payoffs in terms of how you look and feel. Because excess abdominal fat increases health risks, it's especially important for those who accumulate weight in their abdominal area to be diligent to maintain a healthy body weight and prevent future weight gain. For example, Paul, who had a little extra weight in his midsection, started to run, which burns calories and helps shed body fat, and he began to weight train with a daily focus on his abdominal area. And although it was not one specific activity (for example, abdominal crunches) that led to the weight loss he achieved around his midsection, the combination of exercises, paired with eating more high-fiber carbohydrate-rich foods, lean protein, and fewer refined carbohydrates, is what helped get him into the good shape he is in today.

Take a look at some old pictures of your parents, grandparents, and great-grandparents, if possible. Chances are you can see your shape in an ancestor or two. For example, I am pear shaped like my mom; her mother was apple shaped. She was slim until her forties and fifties and then gained weight in her middle. In contrast, my mother's father, was more pear shaped. He was always at a healthy weight, but his brothers and sisters were all quite bottom heavy and all had large thighs that, to some extent, were passed on to my mother and me, much to our chagrin. If you take a good look at all the body shapes in your family, you'll likely see some patterns. My husband and I have many friends with children who resemble them markedly. In our own family, our eight-year-old son, Spencer, is a virtual clone of my husband. He has the same exact body shape as his dad—from his lean arms and legs to his ears and his round bottom. Our four-year-old son, Eli, is more lean than his brother was at the same age, but he shares my hair color at the same age, eye color, and pinky toes.

Inherited Metabolism

Metabolism is the rate at which the body uses energy, or burns calories. The scientist Eric Ravussin of Pennington Biomedical Research Center, in Baton Rouge, Louisiana, has found that the basal metabolic rate—the number of calories we burn just to keep all our basic systems running—varies among us by as much as 500 calories a day. A low or high metabolism can run in families, which suggests genetic involvement in weight control. So yes, you inherit your basic metabolism, but many environmental and nutritional factors affect it, a number of which you can control.

Your hormones, the products of your endocrine glands, are major players in your metabolism. They are the chemical messengers that regulate your body processes and bone structure. Hormones are also important contributors to the shape you are in—inside and out. Excesses or deficits of hormones can lead to obesity. The endocrine system has a basis in heredity, but family eating habits and emotions affect hormonal secretions. If there are conflicts and other stresses in a family, for example, members' adrenal glands can secrete hormones that lead to fluid retention. Women are particularly susceptible to this phenomenon because of their naturally fluctuating hormone levels (see chapter 7 for more about the nutrition needs of women).

No matter what genes you inherited, the ideas and information in this book can benefit both you and your family. Although genetics certainly contribute to your family's various body shapes, many environmental factors influence your body weight and overall lifestyle. It may not be possible for you to change your inherited body structure, but once you take a good look at your own body weight, shape, frame, and medical history and how it relates to members of your entire family, you'll be in a better position to set realistic food and fitness goals (see chapters 2 and 3), make changes in your daily eating and fitness habits, and encourage your family members to do the same in ways that work within their own unique lives.

2

Setting Realistic Food Goals for Your Family

Do French fries and potato chips compose the bulk of your family's vegetable intake? Does your family consider soda and candy as two distinct food groups? Is a cheese, egg, and bacon sandwich with coffee your idea of a balanced meal?

If you answered yes to any of these questions, this book will help you and your family learn how to fit all the foods you love into a healthful, nutritious, and still delicious dietary pattern. You will also learn how to create a home environment that supports your efforts to improve your eating habits. But before you and your family make any changes at all in your food intake, it makes sense to take a look at what, when, and how much you eat, and how your habits are affected by particular challenges you face depending on your age and stage of life.

One Step at a Time

For many of us, it's not too difficult to lose weight. But keeping weight off is what does most of us in. If you're reading this book, it's likely you and your family have not yet found a way to reach your weight-related goals, or perhaps you simply want some guidance on how to incorporate better nutrition into your family life. To achieve this, all of you—even those without significant weight problems—must be ready and willing to make at least some small changes one at a time. Even a small change, like cutting 100 calories a day or eating breakfast each morning, can positively affect your family's food habits. But even if you are successful at making changes individually, it's critical that all family members support one another's efforts (see chapter 4 for tips on how to handle others who may sabotage your ability to achieve and maintain more healthful habits).

So What Are You Eating?

If you truly want to improve your eating habits, one of the best ways to get started is to keep a record of everything that passes your lips for a few days, preferably on two typical weekdays and one typical weekend day. You can use the "Daily Food Log" below to do this; alternatively, you can keep a small notebook in your purse or briefcase or even use your personal digital assistant or your computer to keep track. In addition to recording what you're eating, try to approximate how much you're eating. You can eyeball portion sizes or measure

Daily Food Log		
Time of Day	Food or Beverage	Amount Consumed

them directly. I recommend measuring food at home, at least initially, so that you'll train your eyes to estimate how much you consume. Invest in a clear measuring cup (for liquids), another measuring cup (for solids like cereal, pasta, rice, and beans), a set of measuring spoons (for oils, margarine, salad dressings, and mayonnaise), and a food scale (for meat, poultry, fish, and chicken) to help you see how much you're really eating.

I know this is a time-consuming, demanding effort, but there's really no better way to objectively see:

- What and how much you are eating
- How often you are eating
- What's missing from or lacking in your diet
- What you may be overconsuming

Of course some older teens or even preteen children may *want* to keep track and even have fun doing so, but make sure that it's their choice to keep track, and avoid pressuring them if they choose not to. If they see you make an effort to change your own ways, it may inspire them to pay more attention to their own food intake, and they may even decide to keep tabs on themselves at a later point.

Once you see how you and individual family members currently eat, the next step is to determine the dietary pattern that can help each of you meet your calorie and nutrient needs to achieve and/or maintain a healthy body weight (see chapter 10). Knowing the dietary pattern that's recommended for you will help you see objectively how your current food intake measures up. Are you overdoing refined grains and "extra calories"? Are you skimping on low-fat milk products? Is your diet too meat heavy, or are you simply not eating enough vegetables?

Keep in mind that each family member has unique nutrition needs based on age, height, weight, gender, activity level, and individual variables. For example, having food allergies, diet-related diseases or conditions such as type 2 diabetes, heart disease, hypertension, or high cholesterol, or following a vegan or vegetarian diet all affect food choices. Each family member also has a distinctive lifestyle involving personal temperament, unique food tastes, physical activity preferences, and schedule. Sometimes conflicts that affect food intake arise between family members (see chapter 4 for solutions to some common food-related conflicts). In addition, where each of you is in terms of age and stage in life greatly influences your eating and fitness habits, and subsequently your body weight. Because these factors are so important to consider, chapters 5 through 9 provide individual goals for infants, toddlers, tweens, teens, women, men, and seniors. Specific tips for women, men, boys, and girls to help them manage their weight are provided in these chapters and throughout this book to help you and your entire family improve your nutrition and fitness habits and change your family "weighs"!

3

Making Fitness Fun for Your Family

Does e-mailing and text-messaging friends or channel surfing with a remote control make up most of your physical activity each day? You already know physical activity is good for every member of your family, even those with medical problems. You have heard it over and over again. Regular physical activity not only helps you control your weight and improve your physical appearance, but it benefits your heart and bones and lifts your mood. It also gives you strength and stamina to get up and go, aids digestion, and helps eliminate wastes from the body. With all those positive effects associated with being physically active, why isn't it a priority in your home? What are your excuses?

Excuse One: You Don't Have Time

This is my personal favorite that I use a lot. Many of us feel so time starved. With so much to do and not enough time to do it, it's often easy to justify pushing fitness aside or not making it a priority.

I personally love to exercise and be physically active, but with the clock ticking, two full-time jobs (one working out of the home, one raising two young sons and maintaining a household), it's a miracle I find *any* time for exercise. What do I do to stay fit? I plan for the worst and hope for the best. On Sundays, I take a look at my weekly schedule and make appointments with myself to exercise or simply be physically active. The mornings are always best for me because I like to be efficient and shower only once a day! One or two days a week, I drop my two boys off at school and head straight to the gym. I spend about fifteen to twenty minutes weight training with 5- to 10-pound weights, and thirty minutes walking at 4 miles per hour on a treadmill. On Fridays, I try to make it to a tap dancing class, one of the most enjoyable, challenging, and sweat-inducing activities I have found in a long time. I round out the week with one or two gym workouts on the weekends, depending on what my family has planned.

Also, when my sons were younger, I would push them in their strollers to get them to school twenty-eight blocks away. On my gym days, weather permitting, I'll walk home instead of taking a bus, subway, or taxi. I also walk outside as much as possible during the day to pick up one of my children or run errands. I've also been known by my husband on occasion to plunk down and do twenty or more push-ups (OK, I admit the girlie ones) before bedtime.

As for the rest of my family, they too find time to be active. My husband, Brian, has always been active but has become a gym rat over the last few years. Because he finds it tough to work out midday or at the end of the day (when he likes to get home by seven to spend some quality time with me and our kids), he decided that mornings were best for him. Monday through Thursday, he gets up with the roosters (at about 5:15) and hits the gym, although I much rather him be with us in the morning to lend me a hand. I know he needs to be fit for himself, especially because of his family history of type 2 diabetes. On weekend mornings, he watches the kids so I can hit the gym myself. Brian's claim to fame is that he's run the New York City Marathon three times. He hopes to do another someday when our boys are older and he has more time to train.

As a family, we are extremely active and always on the go. We bowl, ice skate, play softball and basketball in our backyard when the weather is nice on weekends, and my husband and I chase after our two boys who are constantly on the run (they never walk, but run everywhere). Our older son plays organized basketball or baseball on weekend mornings. By their very nature, our boys are always playing and being physically active. They are the opposite of couch potatoes, although they admittedly wind down in the evening with an hour or so of television, and because my husband and I love TV ourselves, we can't deny them this pleasure, in moderation. We purposely do not have any type of system that allows them to play video games, and they don't seem to miss it. We hope that by our example we're helping our boys see that being physically active is important for our muscles, our bodies, and our minds.

So how can you, as an individual, and your family, as a whole, find the time for fitness? With 1,440 minutes in every day, you'd think it would be easy to carve out some time for formal exercise or just some brisk walking. For adults, work demands and family demands leave little time for fitness. Perhaps you feel that whatever project you have at work must come first. Or you're so busy caring for your family—cooking, running a household, and organizing everyone else's life—you leave little time for yourself. Maybe you think about fitness as all or none: if you can't spend an hour at the gym, you may as well skip it. For kids, homework and extracurricular activities (unless they're sports or fitness related) may leave little extra time for much else. Whatever the reasons, it's easy to see that with the many demands in life, time is what many of us feel we lack most. The good news is that you can find the time; any amount of time you spend being active, even ten minutes, can positively impact your health, mind, and body. Setting small achievable goals for physical activity is a great place to start. But before you can set goals, you need to see what you're doing now and where you can find the time you need to be more active.

On a plain piece of paper, in a notebook, on your computer, or on the form (on page 28), keep track of how you spend your time on a typical day. Note how much time you spend on each activity (whether it's sleeping, sitting at a desk doing homework or using a computer, watching television, walking, taking a fitness class, hiking, and any other things you do that day). Keeping track will show you how you usually spend your time and will also help you objectively spend some time to be more physically active, both when you're alone or with other family members. When you see how you and your family members actually spend your time, you may be surprised to find some small windows of opportunity during your day to squeeze in some fitness.

Here's how Carolyn, a busy mother of three, used this form to assess and improve her own activity habits:

As the mother of twin nine-year-old sons and a three-year-old daughter, Carolyn had little time for fitness but really wanted to get back into some sort of fitness routine. As many moms often do, Carolyn had always put her own needs aside to care for her children. Not being fit had taken a toll on her emotionally (she used to relieve stress

How You Spend Your Day	
Time of Day	**Activity**

by taking long walks and listening to music) as well as physically (she often felt winded when she ran errands and still carried around some excess baby weight and missed feeling more toned). See page 29 for how Carolyn filled out her form.

Carolyn found that she had so many domestic obligations to take care of when the kids were at school, she was constantly on the run, carpooling her kids to and from school and other activities, and it wasn't until nighttime, after the kids went to bed, that she would unwind by retreating to her bedroom at 8:30 P.M. to read or watch television. This was the only downtime she felt she had each day, and this mindless time gave her some entertainment and a respite from her hectic day at the same time. She wanted to exercise and found that besides having a playdate with her daughter and her mommy friends, it was tough to find any other time of day to fit in fitness. Because she had not yet lost all her baby weight and knew this was in large part because she wasn't exercising like she used to, she decided she would try to decrease her nightly dose of TV.

Carolyn initially cut fifteen minutes of her nightly TV time and instead filled that time with some gentle stretches, crunches, and push-ups. Then, because she always wanted to do yoga but didn't like to

How You Spend Your Day	
Time of Day	**Activity**
6:00 A.M.	Sleep
6:30–7:15 A.M.	Shower, get dressed
7:15–8:00 A.M.	Make breakfast for family, get kids dressed and ready for school
8:00–9:00 A.M.	Bring twins to bus, drive daughter to school, chat with other moms at school
9:00–11:00 A.M.	Do laundry, make beds, take out the garbage, do other chores
11:00 A.M.–12:45 P.M.	Go grocery shopping, run errands
12:45–1:15 P.M.	Pick up daughter at school
1:15–2:45 P.M.	Have playdate with daughter and her friends
2:45–3:00 P.M.	Twins get home from school
3:00–5:00 P.M.	Clean out backpacks, lunch boxes, make lunch for the next day, watch TV with kids after they do homework
5:00–5:45 P.M.	Give kids baths
5:45–6:40 P.M.	Prepare dinner and have dinner with kids
6:40–7:30 P.M.	Pay bills, check e-mail (my husband is home)
7:30–8:30 P.M.	Put kids to bed
8:30–11:00 P.M.	Read magazines and watch TV in bed
11:00 P.M.–6:30 A.M.	Sleep

take formal exercise classes, she added a thirty-minute yoga video to her routine. She would also put her exercise clothes on two days a week and try to squeeze in a brisk walk (perhaps with another mom) around her neighborhood for twenty or thirty minutes after she dropped her daughter off at school. After several weeks, Carolyn was able to achieve her goals on most days and felt stronger and more energetic, slept better, and felt mentally rejuvenated. She still enjoyed about an hour of television each night but only turned the TV on after she completed her exercise. At the same time she increased her physical activity, she also decided it was time to set more limits on TV and screen time with her kids. She realized her children spent up to four hours total each day watching TV and playing video games. She decided to limit their TV/video time to thirty minutes in the morning (down from an hour—they were early risers) and 1½ hours after school, and only after they finished their homework and baths. And she would also get more fit with them. For thirty minutes after the boys returned home from school, she'd either play hide-and-seek or tag inside or out in the backyard. This gave both Carolyn and her kids more time to be active, and spend more quality time together before the rush to get dinner on the table and the kids to bed.

If you, like Carolyn, analyze how you and your family spend your time, you can find ways to fit more fitness into your day. If, after keeping a log of how you spend your time, you find you spend much of the time talking on the telephone (teenagers are notorious for this), for example, you can pace, take a walk outside, pedal a stationary bike, walk up and down stairs, organize your closet, do dishes, clean your room, do some laundry, or iron some clothes while you talk on the phone instead of simply sitting down. With a little thought and creativity, you can work a little more fitness painlessly into your day.

Excuse Two: You Don't Know Where to Begin

Often the hardest part of any new endeavor is knowing where to start. But you can do it! Now that you've uncovered small windows of time on a typical day during which you can incorporate some more physical activity, it's time to learn how much you need and what types of activities you can realistically pursue. See the table on page 31 to see how much exercise is recommended for you.

If you know you just don't have thirty to ninety minutes to devote to purposeful physical activity in your usual day-to-day life, perhaps you can aim for one or two ten- or fifteen-minute bursts of activity on most days, and try to accumulate more when extra time presents itself such as on weekends or on vacation. Anything is better than nothing when it comes to physical activity; even ten or fifteen minutes of moderate physical activity can help you burn some extra calories, give you energy, and lift your spirits. If you work toward accumulating thirty or more minutes on most or all days, you'll reap even more benefits, but again, some is still better than none.

Now you and your family members are ready to make some choices about the physical activities you are going to pursue. To reap health benefits, it's important to aim for moderate or vigorous physical activities each day that go beyond your usual day-to-day activities (such as walking at a leisurely pace, grocery shopping, doing light household

Getting Physical: How Much Is Enough?		
	If Your Goal Is:	Then You'll Want to Do:
Adults	To reduce the risk of chronic disease and to reduce functional declines associated with aging (goal for older adults)	At least thirty minutes of moderate-intensity physical activity, above usual activity
	To help manage body weight and prevent gradual weight gain	Approximately sixty minutes of moderate- to vigorous-intensity activity (while not exceeding caloric intake requirements)
	To sustain weight loss (if you were previously overweight or obese)	At least sixty to ninety minutes of daily moderate-intensity physical activity* (while not exceeding caloric intake requirements)
Pregnant women	To reduce the risk of chronic disease and to support a healthy pregnancy with appropriate weight gain (see chapter 7)	Thirty minutes or more of moderate-intensity physical activity (barring any medical or obstetric complications); avoid activities with a high risk of falling or abdominal trauma
Breast-feeding women	To reduce the risk of chronic disease and to support healthy weight management postpartum	Same as for all adults; postpartum women can begin or resume moderate levels of exercise anywhere between two and six weeks postpartum (check with obstetrician first); neither acute nor regular exercise adversely affects the mother's ability to breast-feed successfully
Children and adolescents	To reduce the risk of chronic disease and to support optimal growth (height, weight, bone mass, etc.)	At least sixty minutes of physical activity

Source: USDA, Dietary Guidelines for Americans 2005, 6th ed.
*Some people may need to consult with a health-care provider before doing this much physical activity.

chores, or climbing a flight or two of stairs). Here are some examples of both moderate and vigorous activities:

Moderate physical activities:

- Bicycling (less than 10 miles per hour)
- Dancing
- Gardening/doing light yard work
- Golf (walking and carrying clubs)
- Hiking
- Pilates

- Walking briskly (about 3.5 miles per hour)
- Weight training (general light workout)
- Yoga

Vigorous physical activities:

- Aerobic dancing
- Basketball (competitive)
- Bicycling (more than 10 miles per hour)
- Heavy yard work, such as chopping wood
- Running/jogging (5 miles per hour)
- Swimming (freestyle laps)
- Walking very fast (4.5 miles per hour)
- Weight training (vigorous effort)

Activities such as swimming, cycling, and walking can help you maintain cardiovascular fitness (that's the ability of your heart, lungs, and blood vessels to carry blood that contains oxygen to your working muscles) as well as endurance (your ability to do these activities for a prolonged period of time). They are also great in terms of helping your body burn calories and thus manage your weight (see appendix F for approximate calories burned during moderate or vigorous activities.) They may also provide some benefit in terms of muscle and bone health depending on the activity. Weight-bearing exercises— those activities that work against the force of gravity, such as walking, jogging, hiking, climbing stairs, dancing, and some types of weight training—are important to build strong bones, which can help prevent osteoporosis and bone fractures later in life. These activities should certainly be at the core of your fitness regimen, but it's not enough just to do these types of activities. To get the most overall fitness out of your physical activity, you will also want to include resistance or strength training and flexibility training to round out your fitness regime.

Aim for Resistance

Resistance exercise provides so many benefits to all family members at various stages of life. It can help you achieve and maintain muscular strength and endurance, keep your bones strong, and reduce your risk for injury. It can also make simple tasks like lifting groceries, pushing a stroller, or taking the dog for a walk easier. During child-hood and adolescence, building muscle mass can help improve body composition; the more muscle mass, the more efficient the body is at burning calories, which can prevent kids from adding on too much fat mass as they grow. Also, adolescence and young adulthood is the time during which peak bone mass, or maximum bone density, is achieved. It's especially important for kids who are thin, athletic, or those who don't consume enough calcium and vitamin D to find ways to get these key nutrients (see appendix D for food sources of calcium and vitamin D) and, at the same time, increase their bone mass through fitness to reduce their risks for thinning bones or eventual osteoporosis. But keeping muscles and bones strong is not just for kids; doing so through resistance exercise can provide a boon to adults, especially older adults, who lose muscle mass, gain fat mass, and lose bone den-sity with each passing year. Resistance exercise can also promote bal-ance and improve coordination and agility, especially important in older people who may be more prone to falls that can lead to bone breaks and have other detrimental effects on their mobility as well as overall health. Having more muscle mass at any age will not only help speed your metabolism and burn more calories more quickly, but it will improve the appearance of your body, and who wouldn't want that? Resistance training may include using any or all of the follow-ing: free weights (dumbbells or barbells), exercise equipment (for example, a leg press machine), elastic resistance bands, and calisthen-ics, in which you use the weight of your body (to do push-ups, crunches, and squats and lunges, for example). The American College of Sports Medicine recommends two to three weekly sessions of resistance training, and each session should last twenty to sixty min-utes and include at least one set of eight to fifteen repetitions of eight to ten exercises that work all your major muscle groups. See the resources at the end of the book for more information on resistance or strength training.

Flex Those Muscles!

Flexibility training, or stretching, keeps your joints limber and helps you move your body easily whether you're doing formal exercise or just going about your day. Kids are amazingly flexible, and I recall how as a child I was easily able to touch my toes and do splits and back bends in gymnastics class. Being flexible can also help reduce your risk for injury, to which you may be more prone if you're involved in athletics or if you're older. The American College of Sports Medicine recommends two or three 10- to 15-minute sessions a week in which you do four repetitions for each muscle group (ten to thirty seconds per stretch) to provide health benefits. It's important to warm up your muscles before you stretch, so, for example, you can run around with your kids or walk on a treadmill for five minutes to warm up your muscles before you stretch to minimize injury and get the most benefit from your stretches. See the resources at the end of the book for more information about stretching.

Excuse Three: You Find Exercise Boring

Exercise doesn't have to be grueling or boring. If you don't love to go to the gym, you can get physical activity in a variety of ways. Here are some tips to help keep you motivated (and avoid boredom) as you pursue and maintain a more physically active life:

- **Think outside the box.** Exercise does not have to mean sitting on a stationary bike, walking on a treadmill, or lifting weights. Many other activities can be fun and still provide great health and physical benefits. Do you like to go solo or exercise with others? Are sports your idea of fun, or does tap or ballroom dancing or ballet sound more appealing? After years of talking about it, I finally decided to take an adult tap dancing class a few years ago. It's the most rewarding exercise I've ever done. Find an activity that sounds interesting and make a commitment to try it solo or with a friend. If you keep the fun in fitness and look at it less as a chore and more as an opportunity, chances are you'll stick with it long term.

- **Break it down.** Instead of trying to fit in all your exercise in one thirty- to sixty-minute session, why not break it up into shorter intervals (ten to fifteen minutes)? Splitting up exercise into shorter bouts may increase the likelihood that you'll be able to fit it into your hectic day, and it will be just as beneficial to you in terms of health and can also enhance weight loss and produce similar beneficial changes in cardiorespiratory fitness compared with longer, less frequent sessions.

- **Distract yourself.** Listening to music, watching TV, or talking on a cell phone can really help the time pass when you exercise. With iPods, radio headphones, portable TVs, CD players, and books on tape, you have many options. Just be sure to play it safe when you're using these devices, especially when you're outside. If you're walking on a crowded street or wherever cars pass, stay focused on your surroundings and be sure that your music is not so loud that you won't be able to hear oncoming traffic.

- **Team up.** Those who get support from others are more likely to stick with exercise over the long haul. Exercising with a friend, colleague, spouse, child, or significant other is a great excuse to socialize and laugh, and thereby prevent boredom. If you like exercising with a lot of people, you can make friends and stay fit at the same time by joining a walking or running club, a bowling league, or a team sport. Finding activities you enjoy doing with others is a great way to keep exercise fresh and exciting for parents and kids alike.

- **Keep your eye on the prize.** Are you trying to lose weight, build some muscle mass, or reduce stress? If you focus on what's in it for you—all the great benefits exercise will provide—and if you plan something enjoyable to do when you finish your exercise session (such as calling a friend, playing a game, or reading a magazine or newspaper), it may help keep you motivated to move.

Excuse Four: You Have a Medical Condition

If you have a medical condition or physical limitation that makes exercising a challenge, chances are that with the right guidance from your doctor or an experienced certified fitness professional (see the resources at the end of this book), you can follow your own personal fitness plan to help you burn calories, preserve muscle, and derive other benefits that exercise provides. Be sure to speak with a health-care provider before starting any exercise program if you have a chronic health problem such as heart disease, hypertension, diabetes, osteoporosis, or asthma; if you are obese; if you are at high risk for heart disease (if you have a family history of heart disease or stroke, eat a diet high in saturated fat, trans fat, and cholesterol); or if you're a man over the age of forty or a woman over the age of fifty and plan to start vigorous physical activity. Any exercise, even if it's very-low-impact exercise, can provide benefits that will enhance the quality of your life.

Make Fitness a Family Affair

Being active with your family not only helps you reap the benefits of exercise individually, but it gives you a great excuse to have fun with your family and do activities (such as bowling or playing soccer) that perhaps you haven't done since you were a kid. Using the Weekly Family Fitness Goals form on page 38, ask each family member to make a short list of his or her favorite activities. Then decide, as a family, the activities you will enjoy together on at least three days during the upcoming week. Here are some ideas for how you can incorporate fun and fitness with your family:

- Take a brisk walk, run, or bike around your neighborhood, at a local park, or around your kids' track at school.
- Sign up for a charity walk every few months to do with the entire family.
- Play tag, Wiffle ball, soccer, basketball, or softball, or have relay races in your backyard or at a local park.
- Clean your house or wash the car. Give each family member a job, and time everyone to see who can get the job done the fastest (little kids especially love this).
- Instead of driving or taking public transportation, plan to walk somewhere, or get off the bus or train a few stops early just to fit in some extra walking time.
- While watching television, take breaks during commercials to get up off the couch and stretch or do crunches or push-ups.
- Mow the lawn, rake leaves, or shovel snow. Give kids age-appropriate tasks they can do to help you out.
- Plant a garden. Kids love to water plants, and they'll get excited weeks later when they see their flowers bloom or vegetables grow.
- Go on a treasure hunt around the house or in your backyard. Kids love to search for clues, and all the stair climbing or running

to find the treasures will be a challenge, both physically and mentally.

- Set up an obstacle course in your home or your backyard. Inside, you can use pillows, seat cushions, soft balls, sofas, and chairs. Outside, you can use bases (for softball), hula hoops, ropes, pop-up tunnels, and balls. Incorporate different skills like jumping, crawling, hopping, and skipping. Time kids to see how long it takes them to make it through the obstacle course.
- Play catch, kick a ball, throw a Frisbee, or fly a kite in your back-yard, at a local park, or on a beach.
- Instead of your usual movie or other sedentary family activity, pick an activity that requires movement; you can play laser tag, go bowling, play miniature golf, go to a batting cage, hit golf balls, or chase after your kids at a big indoor gym.
- Push a baby or toddler in a stroller (at a pace of about 3 miles per hour).
- Instead of standing on the sidelines, walk up and down the field when you watch your kids play soccer, baseball, or any sport.
- Take the dog for a walk or run, and keep up with your pet!

With a little creativity and planning, even a family member with the busiest schedule can make room for physical activity. Remember to create a schedule that includes a mix of traditional and nontraditional activities, vary your activities (to use different muscle groups and to prevent boredom), and start out slowly. Don't shoot for the stars, but instead think about what you can realistically do as an individual and as a family in any given week. There's nothing worse for your body and spirit than to go gung ho and overdo exercise, only to burn out and not be able to maintain a high level of activity for more than a few weeks or months. Be realistic and gradually build up the time you plan to do certain activities. Add just a few minutes every few days until you can comfortably achieve the minimum of thirty minutes of physical activity (sixty minutes for kids). As the minimum amount becomes easier, gradually increase either the length of time performing an activity or increase the intensity of the activity, or both. Work on making exercise a regular part of your day, regardless of time and intensity. As it becomes a habit, it will become easier to build on your routine and improve everyone's fitness.

Weekly Family Fitness Goals

Family Member	Favorite Activities
_____	_____
_____	_____
_____	_____
_____	_____
_____	_____
_____	_____
_____	_____
_____	_____
_____	_____
_____	_____
_____	_____
_____	_____
_____	_____

Write down at least one activity you will engage in as a family on at least three days this week:

Monday: _____

Tuesday: _____

Wednesday: _____

Thursday: _____

Friday: _____

Saturday: _____

Sunday: _____

Complete the following at the end of the week:

Were you able to achieve your weekly family goals? (circle one)   Yes   No

- If yes, that's terrific! Keep up the good work.
- If no, what could you do differently in the upcoming week to help your family make time to be fit together? _____

4

Overcoming
Food Fights

If we lived in a bubble, it would be relatively easy to set up our individual lives to support our healthy-weight goals. We could buy and prepare the foods we like without having to worry about feeding anyone else. We wouldn't have to worry that others would eat all our peanut butter or devour that special something, not knowing we were saving it for dessert. We wouldn't have temptations like the snack foods or ice cream we buy for our kids staring us in the face or calling our names—we just wouldn't keep those foods in the house. Although this ideal world may come with some benefits (although I must admit I'd miss my husband and kids way too much to subscribe to a life without them, just to save my waistline), living with or frequently interacting with family members during day to day life, on holidays, and in other food-related situations poses many challenges that can undermine individual efforts to maintain a healthy weight.

Each person comes to the table with more than just food on his or her plate. He or she has unique food preferences, ideas about how much or how little to eat, and personal memories and emotions related to food and family meals, all of which interact to create eating and food-related ideas and habits. All of this makes eating as a family a particular challenge.

Following are some common conflicts many families (including my own) face and some solutions for each to help individual family members and the entire family achieve and maintain healthier food-related behaviors to support their weight management efforts.

The Picky Eater

Young children are notorious for being picky eaters. Of course, we want our children to eat a variety of foods to get enough calories and key nutrients to support their growth. However, we need to respect our kids' individual food preferences and try to work healthful foods into their diets in a creative, no-pressure way. Following are some ideas for how to do that.

Ellie is a mother of two young boys: Adam, seven, and Jake, four. Her younger son is very picky when it comes to his food choices. He used to try lots of different foods, including bananas, apples, broccoli, peas, and carrots, but for the last year or so Jake has been more likely to refuse foods, especially fruits and vegetables. Although Ellie, her husband, and older son all eat fruits and vegetables in front of Jake, that alone does not seem to inspire him to eat them.

The solution is to encourage Jake to incorporate at least some fruits and vegetables into his diet. Ellie can offer him a small portion of fruit or vegetables—even just one or two tablespoons—on his plate at each meal. She can even give him some choices and say, "Would you like peas or green beans?" If he refuses, she could say that we always have fruit or vegetables as part of a meal, so even if you don't eat it, it still needs to be on your plate. Although he may only touch or play with his carrots at dinner, or peel but not eat the banana, at least he's being exposed to these nutrient-dense, wholesome foods, and repeated exposure may lead him eventually to consume these foods. To make sure he actually consumes some fruits and vegetables to meet his nutrient needs, she can offer limited amounts of 100% fruit juice such as orange juice (up to 4 to 8 ounces per day) to provide plenty of vitamin C, folate, and other key nutrients, or frozen 100% fruit juice pops made with an ice cube tray and toothpicks. Ellie can also sneak some fruits and vegetables into her kids' meals by adding a mashed banana or natural applesauce into whole-grain pancake and waffle mixes, making sweet potato pancakes or baked sweet potato French fries, or making a smoothie or gelatin with fresh berries. Ellie needs to pay less attention to what her son is not eating, and instead casually tell him that eating fruits, vegetables, and other healthful foods can help keep him feeling strong.

Similarly, Allison often has dinnertime battles with her older daughter, Kelly, age six. Several nights a week, after Allison prepares a healthful meal (for example, baked chicken with rice and green beans), her daughter whines and screams and refuses to eat what's served. Allison doesn't want to force food on her child but is frustrated that Kelly won't even try the food she makes. Allison doesn't want to be a short-order cook and always give Kelly kid food like macaroni and cheese and chicken nuggets, although she does serve these foods at least two or three nights a week.

The solution is for Allison to encourage her daughter to try more foods. Allison can find ways to involve Kelly (time and schedule permitting) in making food choices and preparing dinner. Even if it's just once or twice a week, she can allow her daughter not only to plan out the family meal but help shop for the foods to include. She can also give her daughter age-appropriate jobs such as stirring or mixing, measuring out ingredients, or setting the timer on the oven, and/or setting the table (my son Eli has been setting the table with place mats, napkins, and utensils since he was about three, and he loves it!). Helping choose and prepare a family meal can empower Kelly and perhaps encourage her to taste and even enjoy the food herself. As a backup, when Kelly does not like what's offered, she can prepare her own dinner from some readily available foods such as cereal, low-fat milk, low-fat yogurt, string cheese, peanut butter and whole-grain crackers, and fresh fruits and vegetables. Allison can leave all the utensils, plates, and cups accessible for her daughter, who can then prepare her own spread. That can show Kelly that her mom is not going to prepare multiple dinners, and it also provides a good way to ensure Kelly gets the key nutrients she needs.

The Food Pusher

How many of you have ever said or heard any of these statements in the family in which you grew up or in your own immediate family?

"If you don't eat everything on your plate, you cannot have dessert."

"Have just another bite—you're getting too thin."

"Don't you like my food? I thought it was your favorite. Have a little bit more."

"You will sit here until you finish every last bite!"

I can tell you that no one—I repeat, *no one*—likes to be forced to eat, either directly or in a subtle, passive-aggressive way. Forcing kids to clean their plates may instill a habit that lasts a lifetime, and this can no doubt cause excess calorie consumption, especially when they eat out and are exposed to enormous restaurant portions. It can also limit the foods people are willing to try because they have negative associations with the foods in question. Anna, a young mother, recalls, "I remember when I was a little girl, I hated cooked carrots. The smell, the texture, the taste—horrible! One night at supper my mother forced me to eat a carrot—really forced me. After a few bites, I ran out the front door and threw up. I remember feeling so violated! Being forced to eat something I *knew* would make me sick was just horrible. I understand that my mother was trying to put wholesome food in my body, but it didn't work. I still hate cooked carrots—the smell still makes me nauseated." Melanie, in her thirties, remembers this: "I hated the taste and texture of red meat; I couldn't even swallow it. My parents used to make me sit at the table until it was gone, and they would set a timer until I finished it. I used to pretend to wipe my mouth, but what I really did was spit out the meat. I made sure to throw out the napkins so no one would see what I had done."

Here are some scenarios and solutions to help you and family members overcome food pushing or deal with food pushers.

Scenario: Stephanie grew up in a family with six kids, so it never seemed like enough food was in the house. She is naturally tall and thin and has never had an issue with her weight. She has three kids of her own and takes pleasure in seeing them eat. Stephanie serves food by portioning it out on plates for each family member. When her kids finish everything on their plates, they earn some sort of treat for dessert. Because all of her kids look forward to dessert, they often do clear their plates. Two of her kids are at a healthy body weight, but one of her children—five-year-old Hannah—is big boned and a bit round. Stephanie is concerned, but because she has other children, she doesn't want to single her out in any way at the dinner table.

Solution: Instead of encouraging her kids to clear their plates, Stephanie can serve them, including Hannah, a little less food, and if they are still hungry, encourage them to ask for more. This way they can decide on their own how much they need based on their hunger level and be better able to regulate what they eat as opposed to being enticed to finish what may be too much food. Stephanie can also make it a rule that if they eat about three quarters of what's on their plate, they can have dessert. In my own family, when I don't think my kids have had enough food, I often look at their plates, feel their muscles, and say, "You need three or four more bites to get stronger," which they respond to. Also, Stephanie may want to keep dessert on the table next to their kids' plates so that dessert becomes a regular part of a meal and is not valued more or less than any other item on the table.

Scenario: Linda, her husband, and her eight-year-old son, Jack, have gone to her mother's house for dinner every Sunday night since Jack was a baby. Her mother always makes Linda's favorite comfort foods, among them fried chicken, mashed potatoes, and apple pie. For several months, Linda has been cutting back on what she eats in the hopes of losing the 10 pounds she gained over the last few years. She loves her mother's company and great food, but she dreads Sunday nights because she feels her mother is always staring at her to make sure she eats enough. As a child, Linda always cleaned her plate (but was not forced to—she just did), but now, as an adult, she tries to eat less and takes less of the food offered to her. When Linda tells her mother she's full after about three quarters of a plate of food, her mother makes comments like "What, you don't like my food anymore?" or "How can you eat so little?" or "You're getting too skinny." Her mother clearly takes offense.

Solution: Linda wants to preserve the ritual of going to her mother's home for dinner each week, but at the same time, she does not want to be pressured to eat too much, especially because she's watching her weight. She can talk to her mother, on the phone or in person, before she goes to her mother's home on Sunday nights and explain that she loves her food as much as always but because she's getting older, she needs to eat less at all her meals and would appreciate it if her mother would not comment on how much she is or isn't eating when she's at her house. Linda can also insist (in a nice way) on putting the food on her own plate—she can take less but still aim to eat it all. That way she's cleaning her plate (as she did as a kid) to satisfy her mom but keeps tabs on her portions. She can tell her mother that when she takes less food on her plate, it helps her savor each bite but still get the full enjoyment from the meal.

The Food Cop

Does this sound familiar? Adam, a man in his early thirties who is very muscular but struggles with his weight, recalls, "When I was eleven years old, I was in the kitchen and opened a box of doughnuts that my mother had bought. I had one doughnut—but hadn't asked her if I could. She made me walk two miles each way to the grocery store to replace the entire box of doughnuts, and refused to let my father or older sister drive me there. To this day I give her a hard time for making me do it—first, because it was one doughnut, second, because . . . well, it was one doughnut. Admittedly, I probably knew I wasn't supposed to open the box, but I have basically spent the last twenty years giving my mom grief over this punishment."

If you had a parent like this, there's a chance that you, too, try to control your children's food intake. Or you may take the opposite approach and let your kids have whatever they want. Neither extreme works well. Here are some ideas for how to find some middle ground.

Karen's older son, Steven, age twelve, has always eaten a lot of healthy foods—fruits, vegetables, whole grains, beans, and lean meats. But he also has a sweet tooth (which he inherited from both Karen and her husband). He can't resist any foods that start with C: cakes, cookies, cupcakes, and chocolate. When Steven was younger, he always used to ask permission to take a snack from the pantry, but now that he's older, he helps himself. After school, he usually chooses a snack, and then has dinner, dessert, and a bedtime snack. He has always been at a healthy weight, but lately he's gotten a little thicker around the middle. Because Karen is worried about Steven's weight, she decided to get rid of all the junk in their pantry to help Steven avoid temptations.

Although it can certainly be helpful to keep certain foods—especially snack-type foods that lure us and that we tend to overconsume if they're there—out of the house, banning all sweet indulgences can actually be counterproductive. It may also seem like a punishment to Steven, who may now be more likely to indulge in such foods when he's out with friends or away from home. My mother only occasionally allowed any type of junk food in our house growing up; pretzels and, once in a while, ice cream were about the only real treats we had. Subsequently, I felt very deprived and had a feeding frenzy at my friends' homes during sleepovers (I even remember snacking on not one but two Kit Kat bars, without my mother knowing, at the ice rink during my weekly ice skating lessons).

Karen can allow some snack foods in her home without going overboard. Legalizing these foods, but setting limits on when to eat them (after dinner instead of right after school) and where to eat them (at the dinner table or kitchen counter, and not in front of a TV or computer screen) can help Steven incorporate the snacks he likes without going overboard or craving them even more. She can also encourage Steven to choose his snacks wisely: to buy and keep in the house only the snacks he really likes, instead of wasting calories on foods that don't mean much to him. Because Steven is twelve years old, his daily needs are approximately 1,800 calories; about 200 of those are "extra" calories that he can use to have cookies, candy, soda, or any foods that don't fit neatly into any particular food group (see chapter 10) or any other low-nutrient foods. Chances are Steven is already having more than 200 calories from food such as these that don't neatly fit into any particular food category.

Karen and Steven can, together, come up with some healthy and satisfying snack ideas using foods in the various food categories. Some examples include peanut butter on whole-grain crackers, air-popped popcorn, green apple slices with peanut butter, and trail mix with 2 tablespoons each of dried fruit, nuts, and ½ cup crunchy whole-grain cereal. If Steven consumes a meal pattern similar to that recommended to help him meet his calorie and nutrient needs, he can then spend his 200 extra calories on cookies and other treats without guilt.

The Relentless Ranter

Does this sound familiar? Carrie, a thirty-five-year-old petite woman, recalls, "My parents have basically been on my case since I was a teenager about eating. First, they constantly warned me to be careful about getting fat because I was short and petite. Then, because I've gained a bunch of weight over the past few years, when we eat together they look at me, pat me on the stomach, and politely tell me I've had enough. But now that I'm losing some weight, they warn me not to get too thin. They drive me mad!"

Do you have family members who constantly comment on what you're eating, what you're not eating, how much you're eating, how much you're not eating, how thin you are, or how heavy you're becoming? Do you constantly make these kinds of comments to your own kids, spouse, or parents? Showing concern is one thing, but providing a running commentary on someone else's eating habits can make the other person feel self-conscious or ashamed, angry or violated, and it may even lead them not to want to eat in front of you or to sneak food.

Unless you have a child who is not growing properly or is losing weight (and does not need to) or have other family members who are losing or gaining weight (and don't need to) for no known reason, or you have a parent, a spouse, or a child who has a serious health condition such as uncontrolled type 2 diabetes or has food allergies and needs to follow a more restrictive diet or avoid certain foods, there's no reason to make negative or judgmental comments about what someone else is eating or how they look, period. If you find you are guilty of this (even I, at times, pat my dad on his sometimes enlarged belly and ask, very nicely, "Have you gained weight?"), try to put yourself in the other person's shoes. You'll attract more bees with honey, so if you are truly concerned about someone else, express your concern and ask if you can help in any way. Attacking and putting people on the defensive is the very best way to encourage them to continue harmful or destructive habits and avoid you like the plague, which, in families, can create a problem.

The Sneaky Snacker

Do you find food wrappers or cans of already eaten food under beds or stuffed in a drawer? Sneaking food can be harmless or it can be a sign of disordered eating or an eating disorder. Gloria, a mother of two, is a self-described closet eater and compulsive overeater. She recently revealed the following to me: "When my husband Bill was going to law school at night, I'd get home from work and would feel lonely and hungry. So one night I ordered veal parmesan and garlic bread from my favorite Italian restaurant. As I was eating my ultimate comfort food, I heard Bill's key in the door. Not wanting him to see me eating this, I grabbed the food, still in the tins, and ran into the bedroom. I hid the food under the bed. Little did I realize that our three-month-old pound puppy, Gypsy Rose Lee, smelled the delicious food and bolted under the bed and ate it. Bill kept asking me why he was smelling garlic. I said our neighbors must have ordered in again. Poor Gypsy! When she came out from under the bed, her belly was so blown up I was afraid she'd explode, not to mention she reeked of garlic!"

In Gloria's case, closet eating was certainly a sign of a bigger problem. She later admitted to me that she suffered from bouts of bulimia (which she has subsequently, and with a lot of hard work, successfully overcome). If your child, your spouse, or some other family member seems to be sneaking food, it's best to talk to them but not make food the focus. Without being accusatory, ask them how they are and if they would like to talk about anything. In some cases, you may think someone sneaked food when in fact they just helped themselves without you being there. In other cases, however, sneaking food may be a sign of compulsive overeating or a similar problem. If you suspect your child or spouse may suffer from an eating disorder or may be moving in that direction, you may want to seek professional help for tips on how to handle it. See the resources at the end of the book for more information about eating disorders and who to turn to for help.

Dueling Diets

Perhaps you are at a healthy body weight and eat a relatively balanced diet, but your spouse has decided to go on a diet. Perhaps he now gave up meat and eats a vegetarian-type diet. Maybe he wants just to lose some weight to look better, or maybe this is his response to the higher cholesterol or blood pressure numbers discovered at a recent physical. Now that he is taking some steps to cut back calories, does he expect you to do the same, even if you don't have any issues with your own body weight? Does he get upset when you eat foods he's trying to avoid, or does he try to convert you to eat the way he now does? Or is he simply embarrassing you by his new habits?

When I was a teenager, my mother and three of her friends—four Barbaras in all!—were following a ridiculous diet that said they could eat whatever they wanted during one meal a day as long as they ate the entire meal in an hour. One night, we all went to dinner. I remember the women ordered their dinners and, with their eyes on their watches, managed to devour their entrées, including steak and fish, and huge baked potatoes with butter, and chocolate or cheesecake for dessert. All the husbands, including my dad, my brother, and I sat there mortified as the women finished their desserts well before our entrées were served! Although my mother and her friends now laugh about that night, it was one of those experiences that undoubtedly prompted me to become a registered dietitian in the first place and help others stop the diet insanity once and for all.

If you have a spouse or some other family member who simply wants to eat healthier, be supportive; try not to bring tempting foods in the house purposely, encourage him or her to order dessert if the person really wants to skip it, or undermine verbally by making comments like "I don't know why you're not having the bread—you don't need to lose weight." Try to support their efforts, but also let them know that although you're happy for them and will do your best to support them, you want to eat what you want and you don't want to feel bad about it. When you talk with each other, tell the person how you feel. Say, "I feel . . ." instead of "You make me feel . . ." That will help this person not be on the defensive and understand where you're coming from.

If your child or teenager starts to diet on his or her own, or begins to avoid certain foods or food groups; you notice unnecessary weight loss; you suspect your child is sad; or you hear negative comments about his or her weight, body, or overall appearance, it may be a sign of disordered eating behaviors or an eating disorder. Gently ask your child about his or her thoughts, feelings, and eating habits without being confrontational or accusatory. Ask how you can help with self-esteem and healthy eating. If you suspect your child may have or is on the road to an eating disorder, speak to your physician. See the list of resources at the end of the book.

part two

Achieving and Maintaining a Healthy Weight for Life

5

The Infant, Toddler, and Tween Years

Whether you're a new parent or have been one for quite some time, you know firsthand how quickly children grow, change, and develop. Since there is no one-size-fits-all prescription for how to feed children, this chapter will arm you with information about what makes each age and stage of childhood unique, how to determine your children's unique nutritional needs, and how to help them meet those needs to grow optimally both physically and mentally.

Infants and Toddlers

Who doesn't love to squeeze the cheeks of a chubby baby? The size of a new baby and his or her risk for becoming overweight later in life depends on so many factors including early influences such as maternal eating habits and weight gain during pregnancy, smoking history, and genetics. According to the World Health Organization (WHO), differences in growth rates among infants and children up to age five are more influenced by nutrition, feeding practices, and environment than by genetics or ethnicity. Now, more than ever, overweight is striking more and more young children, including infants, at an alarming rate. In a recent study published in the July 2006 issue of the journal *Obesity*, researchers examined more than 120,000 children under the age of six over a twenty-two year period and found that the prevalence of overweight among the children increased from 6.3 percent to 10 percent (a 59 percent increase); even in the youngest subjects—infants from birth to six months—being at risk for overweight jumped by 59 percent, and being overweight increased by 74 percent. Because many researchers now believe that being overweight at any age, even during infancy, is undesirable, it is more important than ever for parents to take steps to modify their environment to prevent overweight and its many side effects in their offspring.

When you feed your infant, try to follow her cues as much as possible. Never force-feed, and give yourself some time to get to know your baby and identify when she's hungry as opposed to wet, tired, or just plain fussy. I know firsthand it's not always easy to know what your infant wants, but feeding on demand seems to be the best way to meet your infant's nutritional and emotional needs. Every baby has different eating habits, and the best way to judge if a baby is eating enough is to check her diapers. If your infant wets four to six diapers a day, the urine is pale in color, and weight increases at visits to the pediatrician, he or she is likely getting what's needed. Keep in mind that most infants go home from the hospital weighing less than they did at birth but tend to rapidly gain that weight back over the next several days.

Although it is certainly a personal choice whether to breast-feed or bottle-feed, studies suggest that breast-feeding offers children some protection against future obesity. It also seems to decrease the risk for asthma, type 1 and type 2 diabetes, some cancers, and sudden infant death syndrome (SIDS). If you choose to and are able to, breast-feed for as long as you can (see chapter 7 for nutrition goals for breast-feeding). According to the American Academy of Pediatrics, up to one year is the optimal amount of time to breast-feed. If you bottle-feed, discuss with your pediatrician the type of formula you should use. Although iron-fortified formula is typically recommended, some infants may need other types of formulas if they have certain medical conditions or appear to have allergies or intolerances (see the resources at the end of the book).

Whether you breast-feed or bottle-feed (or do some combination of both, as I did), allow your infant to guide his or her intake. Babies grow at enormous speed during their first year of life, in fact, faster than at any other time in life. The average baby triples his or her body weight—or gains about 15 pounds—during the first year of life. Appetite usually coincides with growth, so when growth is rapid, appetite is usually high. But after the first six months, as infants take more interest in their environment and other people, appetite often decreases. This is not necessarily a red flag. As long as your infant and then toddler grows steadily and doesn't fluctuate too greatly when measured by the pediatrician using pediatric growth charts, you can rest assured your child is getting adequate calories to meet his or her needs.

Sometimes, especially when infants' and toddlers' appetites seem to diminish, parents become overly concerned, and to compensate, they may unknowingly (or knowingly) push extra food on their children. Avoid the temptation to force-feed or pressure your child to eat (infants do not need to finish each and every bottle to grow at a healthy rate and get key nutrients they need). A recent study in the journal *Pediatrics* found that mothers who give their infants more control over their attempts to eat solid food are better equipped to regulate their own food intake than those who have mothers who try to control their intake by continuously forcing or offering food, or distracting them so they'll eat.

Because too much weight gain in infancy may be associated with the onset of obesity in childhood and adulthood, teaching infants to eat when hungry and stop when full is a great lesson, one that can only help them later in life when they increasingly make their own decisions about what and how much to consume.

Between the ages of four and six months, you can safely add solid foods to your infant's menu. Infants who sit without support, weigh twice as much as they did when they were born, seem hungry after eight to twelve breast feedings or 32 ounces of formula in a day, and take great interest in what you're eating are likely ready to try some real food. Experts from the American College of Allergy, Asthma, and Immunology recommend that infants at risk for allergies (for example, they have a family history of food allergies), should wait to begin solid foods until six months of age, dairy products until twelve months, hen's eggs until twenty-four months, and peanuts, tree nuts, fish, and seafood until at least thirty-six months. They recommend that infants who do not appear to be at risk for allergies be given solid foods at six months, and that potential allergens, which include eggs, peanuts, tree nuts, fish, and seafood, can be introduced one at a time and with caution. Because wheat and soy foods may also pose an allergy risk, they suggest you speak with your pediatrician to discuss their inclusion in an infant's diet. Page 54 contains some tips to help you feed your under-twos.

Top Tips for Feeding Your Under-Twos

- Take a time-out and turn off the TV. Mealtimes are a great time for you and your child to spend quality time together. Limit distractions as much as possible. This will help your child learn to focus on the food, not get sidelined by too much noise or visual stimulation, and not get used to eating in front of the TV, which can lead to mindless overeating.

- Sit your baby in a high chair near or at the dinner table. Teaching your child to eat at the table as opposed to on the sofa or in the bedroom is a great way not only to keep your house neat but to instill a good habit that can last a lifetime.

- Offer small portions of a variety of nutritious foods, and let your child decide whether or how much to eat. It's not unusual for infants' appetites to fluctuate, so respect them and resist the urge to force them to eat, especially when they start to push food away or spit it out.

- Offer new foods one at a time every two to four days. That can help you identify any food your child may be sensitive to. If you suspect your child has a reaction—such as a rash or a bellyache—in response to a particular food, be sure to check in with your pediatrician. You can offer mixed foods only after you have determined your child is not allergic to the individual ingredients.

- Offer fruit instead of juice. Although small amounts of 100% fruit juices (such as orange juice, cranberry juice, white grape juice, and apple juice) can provide healthful nutrients that infants and toddlers need, encourage fruit instead of juice, especially during the first year in life, to provide fiber and other key nutrients and help children develop a taste for a wide range of fruits. If after age one your child resists fruit, up to 4 ounces of 100% fruit juice a day can provide some nutrients.

- Stay the course. Always keep in mind that babies and young children can be very picky; if they refuse to eat a particular food, they may decide to try it after several exposures, even as many as ten or fifteen. If after a week or two your child still refuses to try something, offer another food in the same category.

If you offer children a variety of healthful foods (whole-grain breads and cereals, fruits, and vegetables), they are much more likely to choose these foods as they get older when they're more in control of what they eat.

Following is a sample menu for a typical child between the ages of one and two:

Sample Menu for a One- to Two-Year-Old Child

A typical child between the ages of one and two requires approximately 900 calories and about 30 to 40 percent of their calories from fat. Here's what 900 calories can look like on a typical day, based on the meal pattern described in chapter 10:

Breakfast
½ cup oatmeal (1 grain)
½ cup sliced strawberries (½ cup fruit)
1 cup whole milk (1 cup milk/yogurt/cheese)

Lunch
1½ ounces grilled chicken, cut in small pieces (1½ ounce meat/beans)
¼ cup mashed sweet potato (¼ cup vegetables)
½ cup whole milk (½ cup milk/yogurt/cheese)

Dinner
½ cup macaroni (1 grain)
1 ounce/slice cheese (70 extra calories)
½ cup peas and carrots (½ cup vegetables)
1 teaspoon trans fat–free margarine (1 oil)

Snacks/Desserts (in between meals)
2 vanilla wafers (32 extra calories)
½ cup natural applesauce (½ cup fruit)

Young Children and Preteens

More and more kids are becoming overweight, with no signs of a slow-down. In just the last six years, the number of children between the ages of two and five at risk of overweight or overweight has increased from 22 percent to 26 percent; the number of six- to eleven-year-olds considered at risk or overweight has increased from about 30 percent to 37 percent.

There are multiple reasons why so many kids today are overweight. The availability of highly palatable high-calorie, low-nutrient foods such as fast food, soda, and candy, lack of opportunities in school and at home to be more physically active, and a genetic predisposition to overweight are all contributors. On the family front, having an overweight mother greatly increases a child's chances of becoming obese (see the box "Overweight Mom = Overweight Child?" on this page). Having two overweight parents can also increase the risk. Being overweight tends to run in families because of genetic and environmental similarities, so it's important to make achieving and maintaining a healthy weight a family affair instead of just an individual effort.

As you probably know all too well, kids often have some distinct eating habits. Many are overly particular about their food choices; others eat everything in sight. Case in point is my two sons. My older son, Spencer, loves fruits and vegetables, but my son Eli won't touch them unless I sneak them in some foods (for example, put mashed banana or natural applesauce in pancakes or add shredded carrots to chicken meatballs). Some kids refuse to try new foods or eat any foods mixed with or touching other foods.

Although it may be quite frustrating, it's critical to respect your child's personal food preferences, provide a wide range of healthy foods and beverages, and allow your child some choices at meal and

Overweight Mom = Overweight Child?

Did you know that by age six, children of overweight mothers are fifteen times more likely to be obese than children of lean mothers? Researchers at the Children's Hospital of Philadelphia and the University of Pennsylvania followed seventy children for six years. Thirty-three of the children had overweight mothers, and thirty-seven had lean mothers. Those children with overweight mothers weighed more than those with lean mothers by age four, and weighed more and had more body fat by age six. They found dramatic increases in body fat, especially between ages three and six, and the researchers believe that some genes involved in body weight may become activated at this time. Only 1 in 37 of those with lean moms was overweight. The researchers suggest that overweight prevention efforts should begin by age four.

Source: R. I. Berkowitz, et al, "Growth of children at high risk of obesity during the first six years of life: implications for prevention," American Journal of Clinical Nutrition 81, no. 1 (2005): 140–46.

snack times. Try to involve them as much as possible in food shopping or meal preparation. Kids, especially young ones, love to stir and mix things, so when you have the time (not, for example, during the morning rush, but perhaps at dinnertime on a Friday night), encourage your kids to participate in not only choosing the menu but cooking or preparing food. This activity will increase their willingness to try the food they had a hand in creating.

Also, and perhaps most important, try to model the healthy food choices and eating habits you want to see in your kids. Eat in front of them and show them you practice what you preach. Although it's challenging, you want to find a balance between encouraging healthy habits and empowering kids to make their own food choices so they eat enough and teaching your kids to get enough calories from food to meet their needs for growth and development while not exceeding their needs and promoting too rapid or unhealthy weight gain. If you have many children, with different body types, it can be quite a challenge to feed your family. But with the help of this book, and by looking at each family member as a unique individual with his or her own personal needs, you can do it. See chapter 4 to learn how to manage family conflicts that get in the way of healthy eating.

Calorie Goals

Calorie needs for kids differ based on age, gender, and activity level. Here are some estimates of how many calories typical children and preteens need to manage their weight based on a sedentary activity level. Those who are more physically active and/or play sports can likely afford more calories and still maintain a healthy body weight. (See chapter 10 to find the suggested food patterns for each calorie level.)

	Age	Calories per Day
Girls	2–3	1,000
	4–7	1,200
	8–10	1,400
	11–12	1,600
Boys	2–3	1,000
	4–5	1,200
	6–8	1,400
	9–10	1,600
	11–12	1,800

Nutritional Goals

In general, children tend to miss out on many of the key nutrients they need for optimal growth because they usually have low or limited intakes of fruits and vegetables (high in fiber, antioxidants, and nutrients including vitamin A, vitamin C, folate, and potassium) as well as fish (high in omega-3 fats, which play a key role in cognitive growth and development). Kids' diets tend to be snack heavy. Approximately 25 percent of kids' diets come from sugary snacks including soda, fruit drinks, candy, and cookies. Also, as kids get older, they increasingly make more choices about what to eat, especially when they're at school or with friends. But parents can use the following strategies to help kids meet their nutritional needs, support their growth, and encourage a healthy body weight as they mature:

- **Limit where the family eats.** Make it a rule that your family eats at the table or kitchen counter. Just as when your kids were infants, it's more important now than ever before to set some ground rules, not only to provide some structure but to instill healthful habits. Eating in the kitchen and only in the kitchen is a great way to avoid mindless munching that may occur while you or your family watch TV, work on a computer, talk on the phone, or play video games.

- **Make a milk switch.** At the age of two, begin to make the switch from whole milk to low-fat or skim milk, low-fat or nonfat yogurt, and low-fat cheese. Because dairy products are notorious for their high-fat, saturated fat, and cholesterol content but at the same time are invaluable sources of calcium and other key nutrients, switching to low-fat options can help children get all the nutritional benefits with fewer calories.

- **Limit liquid calories.** It's a good idea to help your kids not even get started on soda, fruit drinks, or any sugary beverages (with the exception of 100% fruit juice). These drinks are often loaded with calories and have few nutrients, if any. Drinking too many calories can potentially displace more nutritious beverages such as low-fat milk and water in the diet or leave less room for more nutrient-dense foods. Although I drink diet soda myself and occasionally bring it home, I do not buy sugary soda or drinks, and fortunately, both my sons seem to be happy with mostly low-fat milk and water. If your kids are already hooked on soda and other sugary drinks, slowly remove them, one by one, from the house, and replace them with low-calorie or noncaloric beverages including water and seltzer with fresh fruit slices or a splash of 100% fruit juice. It's up to you if you want to offer diet soda. In moderate amounts (a few cans a week), there may be no harm, but some evidence indicates it can weaken children's bones and have other negative health effects. I do drink it myself but have never offered it to my children, and they do not seem to want it, nor have they ever tasted it. Encourage your children to choose alternatives such as seltzer with some lemon or lime; if they still want soda, encourage them to drink no more than one 12-ounce can every few days if not less often and to make it a special treat (for example, when they go out to dinner) instead of a daily indulgence.

- **Choose fruit over juice.** Although 100% fruit juice such as orange juice, cranberry juice, white grape juice, and apple juice can provide some beneficial nutrients and antioxidants, it often lacks fiber, which fills you up, and is quite easy to overconsume. Portions of 4 to 8 ounces can fit into any healthy eating plan, but encourage your kids always to go for fruit first, and have juice on special occasions (for example, at birthday parties). If they're already juice junkies, you can dilute the juice or serve it in smaller cups until they no longer exceed 8 ounces per day.

- **Consume some protein at each meal.** Protein can support adequate growth and repair of muscles and other body tissues, and it provides energy. Protein-rich foods including foods from the meat/beans and milk/cheese/yogurt food categories and, to a lesser extent, those in the grains and vegetables food categories, can fill kids up and provide them with other key nutrients such as B vitamins, iron, zinc, and in some cases, calcium and fiber, to meet their needs. See chapter 10 for a complete description of each key food category.

- **Teach smart snack habits.** In-between-meal snacks can help fill some nutritional voids left from mealtimes. Because kids are constantly growing, snacking is a common ritual. When your kids are young, instead of automatically offering typical snack foods that are often devoid of nutrients, choose foods from the key food groups as recommended in chapter 10. Some great snack options include whole-grain crackers with cheese, low-fat yogurt, fresh fruit, vegetable slices dipped in low-fat salad dressing or salsa, and air-popped popcorn sprinkled with grated cheese. When it comes to cookies, candy, and other low-nutrient, high-sugar snack foods, teach your kids that they have a certain number of extra calories to play with each day and to choose those calories wisely. My older son, for example, definitely inherited my sweet tooth; I always tell him he can choose as many snacks as he wants from the refrigerator (fruit, vegetables, low-fat yogurt, and cheese), but he needs to limit snacks from the pantry to about 150 calories a day (that's equal to one granola bar, three cookies, or two cookies plus one small package of fruit snacks). I also teach him to save what he wants for dessert and choose more healthful foods as in-between-meal snacks.

- **Emphasize what's in it for them.** As you teach your kids to make their own decisions about what to eat, do so in ways they can relate to. Instead of saying, "If you eat too many cookies, you'll get fat," say, "It's OK to have one or two cookies, but having a big banana can help give you the energy you need to run faster or hit the ball farther in Little League." Speaking in positive terms and emphasizing the potential benefits they may derive from making more nutritious food picks can potentially help kids choose their foods and the amounts they consume more wisely.

Exercise Goals

Children currently do not get the recommended sixty minutes of physical activity each day, and at the same time, they spend anywhere between three and five hours each day playing computer or video games, watching television, or some combination. Although more research is needed, some evidence indicates that simply encouraging more daily physical activity in children can reduce overweight. At home, setting limits on leisure time spent watching TV or playing computer/video games to no more than two hours a day is one way to help reduce sedentary behavior and find some more time for kids to be physically active. My two sons are very physically active. It seems they run everywhere and spend a lot of their playtime wrestling, playing ball, or engaging in other active pursuits. They do watch TV but mainly during the half hour just before dinner and perhaps another half hour before bed. One way to limit TV/computer/video game time is not to have televisions or computers in your kids' bedrooms but instead to have them (if you choose) in a more central place in your home.

Kids spend many waking hours at school, and unfortunately, few offer regular gym classes or periods during which kids can be physically active. As your kids get older, they'll have many opportunities to engage in organized sports, which can help them incorporate more daily physical activity and teach them great athletic and social skills. You can gently encourage your children to find activities they enjoy; if they are resistant, do not force them to participate. Simply try to help them find ways to be more active, either with you or one or two of their friends. See chapter 3 for tips and ideas to help your kids incorporate more fitness into their daily lives.

6

Teenagers

Today's teens have more independence than ever before. They are much more in control of what they wear, where they go, and how they spend their time. Because they have so much more autonomy, they make a lot more decisions that affect their body weight and overall health. They live in a world in which highly palatable low-nutrient foods are available 24/7, and technology—cell phones, pagers, and computer screens—provide them with practically anything they want, whenever they want, with just the press of a button. Most teens seem to care little about their present or long-term health. Many teen girls do care about being thin and lean, whereas many teen boys strive to be buff and in great shape athletically.

Growing, Growing, Gone!

Becoming a teenager is marked by dramatic changes in body shape and size. There are rapid periods of growth (often characterized by increased appetite), and nutrient and calorie needs are typically higher during the teen years than at any other time in life to support growth, especially bone growth. Three out of four teens, despite their concerns, are destined to become overweight as adults. Consider this:

- The average fifteen-year-old girl today weighs ten pounds more than she did in 1963 at the same height; similarly, the average fifteen-year-old boy weighs 15 pounds more and is only an inch taller than he was in 1963.
- Since the 1960s, the rate of obesity among teens has tripled, and there are no signs of a slowdown; in the last six years alone, those twelve to nineteen years of age who are at risk for overweight or presently are overweight increased from 30 to more than 34 percent; the prevalence of overweight in this same population increased from 15 to more than 17 percent.

So why are more and more teens overweight? Research suggests several contributors. Following are a few.

Life in the Fast-Food Lane

Teens are notorious for eating at fast-food restaurants. On a typical day, almost a third of U.S. children and adolescents eat fast food, which is served in larger portions than ever before. In addition to hamburgers, hot dogs, French fries, and pizza, teens are now likely to indulge in more adult decadent coffee beverages. A 12- or 16-ounce coffee drink can have as many as 500 or 600 calories (and lots of fat calories) that can easily add up to excess weight when it becomes a habit as opposed to an occasional treat.

Too Many Snack Attacks

Because many teens skip breakfast or other meals, or live an on-the-go lifestyle, they increasingly rely on snacks to get a quick boost of energy and relieve hunger pangs. Snacking usually occurs during school or after school, at home or in a car, or in front of the TV or computer screen. National data indicate that boys and girls between the ages of twelve and seventeen get about 20 percent of their calories from added sweeteners. A major source of added sweeteners is soda, which makes up more than 10 percent of total calorie intake of U.S. children between the ages of thirteen and eighteen. With approximately 150 calories, and about 10 teaspoons of sugar for every 12-ounce can, soda provides calories and few nutrients and can not only displace calories that could be obtained from more healthful foods but can contribute to excess calorie consumption and subsequent weight gain in teens. Of course, soda is not the only villain. Other foods that are among the top-ten sources of calories in kids' diets include cakes, cookies, and doughnuts, also high in calories and sugar and low in nutrients. With so many tempting foods that are convenient to eat on the run, it's easy to see why so many teens take in more calories than they need and subsequently become overweight.

Fewer Family Meals

When I grew up, we ate as a family almost every weeknight. My mom had dinner on the table by 5:15 P.M., shortly after my dad arrived home from work and we got home from after-school activities. We would congregate at our table, usually filled with good home-cooked food, and talk about our day. For many of today's families, those days are long gone. I make it a priority to have dinner with my two young sons on most weeknights, but my husband usually can't join us because he doesn't get home until about 7 P.M. My sons go to bed by 8 or 8:30, so I like to feed them on the early side. We do eat as a family on Friday and Sunday nights, but because of work and other commitments it's tough to have us all sit down together for a meal on most nights. Today's teens are more likely than younger children to miss family meals because they have much more autonomy and are more able to come and go as they please. After-school activities, study groups, or just hanging out with friends can often mean fewer family meals for teens.

Eating as a family provides parents and kids with a great opportunity to interact and reconnect, and it also gives parents a chance to know what their kids are consuming, provide healthful food and beverage options, and model healthy eating. Studies show that teens who eat with their families eat a more healthful diet, and they may also be less at risk for unhealthy weight-control habits. Although time is tight and schedules are busy, finding at least three nights a week to dine as a family—a good family goal—can not only improve communication among family members but can also improve eating habits.

More Weight Watching

Although dieting is common in adolescents, especially in girls (or boys who want to make weight for a specific sport such as wrestling), it can be counterproductive and quite harmful and should be discouraged. Several studies suggest that dieting can not only increase teens' risks for becoming obese, but it can contribute to the development of disordered eating habits (such as binge eating), full-blown eating disorders (see the box "To Diet or Not to Diet" below), or other harmful behaviors. An increasing problem is the abuse of so-called diet pills to lose weight or steroids to bulk up; both are serious dangers to teen health. For more information, contact the National Eating Disorders Association listed in the resources at the end of the book.

Even moderate dieting among teens increases the risk for developing an eating disorder fivefold. Dieting in teens and children in general should be discouraged, and instead, teens should be encouraged to consume regular meals and snacks that provide key nutrients and an appropriate number of calories to support proper growth and development, engage in regular daily physical activities that are enjoyable and sustainable, and find ways to feel good about their unique body shapes and sizes. See chapter 10, the exercise tips in chapter 3, and the resources at the end of the book to support healthy weight management in teens.

To Diet or Not to Diet

Many teens may diet, fast, skip meals, make themselves vomit, or take diuretics, diet pills, or laxatives to lose weight, but doing so can actually backfire and lead to future weight gain and eating disorders. A recent study of adolescents found that after five years, dieting or engaging in unhealthy weight-control behaviors (as just listed) were not effective in helping them lose weight or maintain weight and actually increased their risks for disordered eating as well as full-blown eating disorders. Even moderate dieting increases the risk for developing an eating disorder fivefold. So teach your teens to feel good about themselves whatever their shapes and sizes, and to engage in positive behaviors to promote a healthy weight (and derive other benefits as well). Consuming a more healthful dietary pattern as recommended in chapter 10 and fitting more regular physical activity into their day (see chapter 3) can provide a good start.

Sources: D. Neumark-Sztainer, et al., "Obesity, disordered eating and eating disorders in a longitudinal study of adolescents: how do dieters fare 5 years later?" Journal of the American Dietetic Association *106, no. 4 (2006): 559–67.*

Brain Freeze

We all know that teens spend considerable time playing video games, watching television, or text-messaging friends or playing games (or even watching TV!) on their cell phones. Teens today are armed with so much technology, they don't even need to go to the library for homework help. Research has shown that the more TV children watch, the more likely they are to be overweight. That makes perfect sense because the time kids spend watching TV is time not spent in more active pursuits (like running around or playing ball with friends). Also, watching TV exposes kids to countless advertisements for high-calorie, high-fat, high-sugar food and fast food, and because many kids snack while they watch TV, that can lead to mindless overconsumption of calories. The Centers for Disease Control and Prevention (CDC) estimates that about 38 percent of teens watch TV for three hours or more each school night. It's a great idea for parents to limit both TV time as well as nonhomework computer screen time to no more than two hours a day.

Too Little Exercise

Teens are always on the go, but they're not always on the move. Of course many teens do participate in after-school sports and other pursuits that keep them active. But unfortunately, many schools today don't offer physical education classes. In 2003, only 28 percent of U.S. high school students attended a daily physical education class according to the CDC. So naturally, teens have fewer opportunities to fit in fitness during the day. The new Dietary Guidelines for Americans recommend sixty minutes of moderate physical activity for kids on most days of the week; currently, among ninth through twelfth graders, more than 1 out of 3 teens did not participate in more than thirty minutes of moderate activity on five or more of the previous seven days or more than twenty minutes of vigorous physical activity on three or more of the prior seven days. Some research even suggests that increasing physical activity alone may be the most effective way to reduce overweight in children and adolescents. Research also suggests that achieving personal fulfillment—not succumbing to pressures from friends or parents or wanting to lose weight—may be the strongest predictor of physical activity in teens. Helping teens find fun activities that can help them boost their skills is one way parents can encourage physical fitness in their kids (see chapter 3 for more exercise tips).

Goals for Teens

It's clear that teens face many challenges that can lead to less than healthy habits and unhealthy weight gain. Parents should certainly be aware of their teens' eating and activity habits, but they should not weigh their teens or do anything to make them self-conscious about their bodies. Parents do, however, want to pay attention to any major weight fluctuations they observe in their teens (which can be a red flag for an eating disorder) and gently encourage and model healthier habits to help their children maintain their weight or slow their rate of weight gain if they are already overweight (and therefore "grow into their weight" as they get taller).

Of course, when we talk about family weight management, the focus is mostly on how to help various family members achieve and maintain a healthier body weight. Many teens are currently overweight, but even those considered at a healthy body weight may also be at risk for developing disordered eating or eating disorders (see the resources at the back of the book for more information if you suspect your teen has or may develop an eating disorder). And although they're more prevalent in girls, eating disorders can also occur in boys.

When I was a teen, I remember far too well how my own weight was on the top of my mind. I remember I had a picture of Madonna with her perfect body hung on the wall in my room. I would stare at that picture and pray that someday, with enough minutes accrued on my portable mini-trampoline and enough bites of food left on my plate at each meal, that I, too, would look like that. I'm proud to say that although I never quite achieved (or came close to achieving) Madonna's exceptional physique, I have lost a significant amount of weight since high school (close to 30 pounds) and have been able to maintain a healthy weight *for me* for many years. And although now I seldom think much about my weight, growing up I probably thought more about my weight, shape, and size than anything else (except maybe boys!).

Just as I did as a teenager, many teen girls today go on diets or take other steps (not always healthful ones) to try to lose weight in an attempt to achieve the thin and fit ideal perpetuated by the media. That's because girls especially learn from an early age that body weight and being thin are important. They learn this not just from images on ads, billboards, television, and movie screens but from what they see and hear at home. A recent study of twelve- to eighteen-year-old teen boys and girls and their mothers found that more girls (33 percent, or 1 in 3) than boys (8 percent) thought more often about their weight and wanting to be thinner. Fifty-four percent of the mothers surveyed said they frequently thought about wanting to be thinner. Compared with girls who accurately perceived that their weight or being thin was not important to their mothers, those girls who thought their mothers wanted them to be thin (whether or not that was true) were significantly more likely to think about wanting to be thinner and to be frequent dieters.

With many boys on wrestling or competitive sports teams that require them to weigh a certain amount, some, at one time or another, may do things to lose weight rapidly, such as use a steam room or sauna to sweat off calories, go on a low- or no-calorie diet to make weight, or engage in other harmful practices that can leave them dehydrated and malnourished, and potentially lead to *very* serious problems.

Teen Calorie and Nutrient Needs

Following are estimates of calorie needs for teen girls and boys, assuming a low level of physical activity. As you can see, boys need about 20 percent more calories than girls. Teens who engage in regular physical activity through sports or other pursuits may need more calories to maintain a healthy body weight as they grow.

See chapter 10 to determine the appropriate menu pattern that matches each suggested calorie level.

Because calorie needs increase in girls when they become teens, they require more nutrients. Calcium needs remain high to support optimal bone growth (see appendix D for food sources of calcium). Iron needs

	Age	Calories per Day
Girls	13	1,600
	14–18	1,800
	19	2,000
Boys	13–14	2,000
	15	2,200
	16–18	2,400
	19	2,600

also increase in both girls and boys. Girls need more iron to replace losses that occur during menstruation (if your child menstruates before the age of thirteen, her iron needs will go up accordingly); boys need additional iron to support increases in lean muscle tissue that occur at this time. (See appendix D for a list of iron-rich foods.)

It's not easy to always have healthful habits when you're a teen. The trials and tribulations (hormonal and otherwise) of just growing up can affect teen eating and fitness habits. Parents can help their teens by being nonjudgmental, setting limits, and choosing their battles. It's tricky to do, but parents need to find ways to communicate positive food and health messages to their teens and resist the urge to express negativity about themselves and their own body weight. A recent study in the journal *Pediatrics* found that girls whose families criticized their weight or made even occasional comments about their weight or eating habits develop lasting problems with body image and self-esteem. If you, as a parent, worry that your teenager is harming himself or herself, seek support from others including health professionals as well as people close to your child (for example, a guidance counselor or teacher). You can help your teens practice independence and make their own decisions and at the same time provide them with tools and opportunities to help them along the way.

7

Women

Someone once said that a diet is something you went off yesterday—or expect to start tomorrow. Although this book is not a diet book, but rather promotes long-term weight management for the entire family, it acknowledges the fact that women may find achieving and maintaining a healthier body weight a daunting task. After all, women need to deal with menstruation, pregnancy and childbirth, and menopause, which all affect their body composition and body weight, not to mention the many life demands they have on their plates.

The Reality for Women

The average mature woman now weighs 24 pounds more and is an inch taller than in 1960; she also weighs in at 164 pounds and stands five feet four compared with 140 pounds and five feet three. That's no surprise given the fact that, on average, women consume 335 more calories each day than they did just three decades ago, mostly in the form of refined carbohydrates or sugary beverages. In the United States, an estimated 62 percent of women, ages twenty to seventy-four, are currently overweight, and about half of that population is obese. The good news is that for the first time in decades, it seems that the rate of obesity and overweight among women has leveled off; no significant increase in incidence of either obesity or overweight occurred between 1999 and 2004, according to the most recent National Health and Nutrition Examination Survey.

So what makes women put on the pounds? Although genetics certainly play a role, many environmental factors contribute to a woman's body weight. Among the factors are:

- Family demands
- Hormones
- Lack of sleep
- Skipping exercise
- Society's expectations

Family Demands—Too Many Things to Do

Superwoman syndrome—doing as much as you can as quickly as you can—causes many women to pack on weight. Are you so overcommitted to career, family, friends, and/or your community that you pay little attention to yourself? The everyday pressures of family life—having one or more children to feed and care for, being involved in your kids' school or after-school activities, working outside the home, and/or taking care of older parents—can certainly have a negative effect on your eating and fitness habits. Having less time to get things done and more responsibilities may lead you to skip meals, mindlessly munch, eat on the run, or emotionally overeat. (Of course, as a mother of two small boys who runs around each day from 6:30 A.M. to 8:30 P.M., it is tough, even for me, to always make the healthiest food choices.) Perhaps the emotional and physical trials and tribulations of motherhood cause you to seek out highly palatable comfort food, such as ice cream or cookies, when you're not even hungry, a habit that can lead you to overdo your calorie intake and put on the pounds.

Hormonal Ups and Downs

Cyclic fluctuations or shifts in hormones can contribute to cravings for sweet, high-carbohydrate, high-fat foods such as chocolate, cookies, ice cream, pasta, and bread. If eaten in excess, these foods can increase your calorie intake and cause weight gain. Menopause usually causes estrogen levels to fall, and for many women, this can lead to increased food intake and weight gain. Several studies also show that during menopause, the weight women tend to gain goes mainly to their abdominal area, and belly fat is associated with an increased risk for type 2 diabetes, high blood fats, high blood pressure, certain cancers, and cardiovascular disease. Hormone therapy, antidepressants, and medications for diabetes and other conditions can contribute to weight gain as well.

Not Enough Zs

Lack of sleep, over time, may affect body weight by increasing appetite, which can lead to weight gain. Researchers believe that chronic sleep loss can cause levels of leptin (a hormone that decreases appetite) to go down and levels of grehlin (a hormone that boosts appetite) to go up. Women who work long hours and/or have children are familiar with sleep deprivation. I know I am! Since my pregnancies with each of my children, my sleep has never been the same. I sleep much more lightly than I used to, and at times my sleep is interrupted late at night or early in the morning by one or both of my kids. It's no surprise that getting less sleep on a regular basis can make you turn to highly accessible, no-fuss convenience or take-out foods at mealtimes or to seek out high-calorie comfort foods such as ice cream late at night once the kids have gone to bed.

Exercise Skippers

Too pooped to move? According to the CDC, in 2003, only 44 percent of women achieved at least thirty minutes a day—the recommended amount of exercise. Forty percent do less than thirty minutes a day, and the remainder are considered inactive. Why are they not exercising enough? A recent study found, not surprisingly, that time pressures, coupled with lack of motivation, prevent many women from getting regular exercise. In this survey of 120 women ages thirty-five to sixty, 59 percent blamed their lack of active time on family commitments, and almost as many said laziness was their excuse. Half the women reported that with more encouragement to make lifestyle changes, they might be able to exercise more. For tips on how to find time to exercise, see chapter 3.

Living Up to Societal Ideals

It's no surprise that many women tend to feel pressure to achieve a perfect, thin, firm, and strong body. Even those who are already at a healthy body weight repeatedly go on and off diets. Reducing calorie intake too dramatically can slow down the metabolism, reduce energy levels, and set women up for nutritional imbalances or deficiencies. It can also lead to or worsen feelings of inadequacy when women resume a more normal dietary pattern. Constant dieting can also adversely affect other family members, especially children, who are highly impressionable and may copy some of the food-related behaviors they see in their parents, their mothers in particular.

So What's a Woman to Do?

Make sure to put yourself on your to-do list; make an appointment with yourself to exercise, take a nap, get a massage, or even prepare a healthy meal just for yourself. Following are some goals and tips to help you on your way toward a healthier weight.

Calorie Goals

Adult women who want to maintain their current body weight need approximately 1,600 to 2,000 calories a day, assuming a low level of physical activity. If you currently consume this amount but need to lose some weight, be sure not to go much below 1,400 calories per day to allow yourself adequate nutrients. Also step up your physical activity. Although each woman is unique, here are ballpark estimates for daily calorie intake for weight management for women of different ages:

Age	Calories per Day
19–25	About 2,000
26–50	About 1,800
51 and above	About 1,600

As you can see, calorie needs decrease with age to compensate for the slower metabolism and decline in muscle mass that occur as we get older. The good news is that if you currently exercise often or maintain a high level of activity, or if you find ways to increase the amount and/or intensity of physical activity you do, you can afford to consume more calories than allotted in chapter 10 to at least maintain your current body weight. Because women need fewer calories than men, we must make every calorie count and incorporate many wholesome, nutrient-dense foods to stay energized and age gracefully. See chapter 10 to find the dietary pattern using all the key food groups that's right for you.

Nutrient Goals

Because our calorie allotment declines as we get older, we must get the most nutrients from the foods we consume. Many women don't get enough iron, a mineral that's important for energy metabolism, brain development, and immune function. Women who may become pregnant or are in early pregnancy need extra folic acid, a B vitamin that reduces the risk of neural tube defects that can cause improper brain and spinal cord development in offspring. Other key nutrients women don't often get enough of each day include vitamin A, vitamin C, vitamin E, calcium, folate, magnesium, potassium, and fiber. (See appendix D for women's needs of and food sources of these key nutrients.)

Fitness Goals

Aim for at least thirty minutes a day (you may need even more to help you keep off any weight you've already lost). If you don't have thirty continuous minutes to invest, break it down into ten-minute intervals. You can walk instead of ride to work, push your baby stroller a little faster, plan for an active weekend outing, such as a bike ride or run with family or friends, or stretch out and do some simple push-ups or crunches on your bedroom floor before bedtime or when your child is taking a nap. Squeeze the fitness in when you can, and pencil in when you'll do this as you would any other appointment. See Chapter 3 for more tips and ideas for how realistically to expend more calories than you do now through physical activity.

Relaxation Goals

If you are able to, set aside one weekday a month to focus just on yourself; if that's not possible, try to take some time each day—even as little as thirty minutes—to take care of yourself and do whatever helps you clear your head and rejuvenate your spirit. Curling up on a sofa with a magazine, taking a bubble bath, or having a twenty-minute nap are some of my favorite ways to unwind and take a mental break during the day. On weekdays and weekends, try to go to bed the same time every night and wake the same time every morning to better regulate your sleep patterns. I know that's easier said then done, especially when you have kids who have uneven sleep habits themselves and you so long for that weekend morning to sleep in. But to have more energy throughout the day, researchers believe sticking to a regular sleep pattern and avoiding alcohol and caffeine two or three hours before bedtime will help you feel more alert and energetic and get things done. A twenty-minute nap can also recharge you midday, so try to sneak those siestas in when the opportunity strikes.

If You Are Pregnant

Stress, fatigue, and food cravings or intolerances may lead you to change your eating habits while you are pregnant. Having been a little bit overweight most of my life, both of my pregnancies with my sons presented me with weight challenges. Could I gain enough but not too much weight to support a healthy pregnancy and still get my body back? Many pregnant women worry that they'll gain too much weight or won't be able to drop the excess poundage after the baby is born. The key is to eat as healthfully as you can tolerate, stay as physically active as you can, and try to consume enough extra calories to gain an appropriate amount of weight during your pregnancy. If you give yourself some time and pay attention to what you eat and start to be more physically active after your baby is born and once your obstetrician gives the okay, you should be able to lose all the weight you gained.

Unlike many celebrity moms or others who miraculously go home from the hospital in their jeans or resume their prepregnancy weight within weeks of giving birth, most of us mortals need some extra time to take off the weight. Of course if you gain a lot of weight when you're pregnant, it will likely take longer and be tougher to take all the weight off, especially with all the new demands on your time and emotions. And with each pregnancy, it becomes more difficult to lose excess weight, especially if you kept a few pounds on from a previous pregnancy. With my first son, it took me about five or six months postpartum to lose the 23 pounds I had gained; I even ended up weighing about 2 pounds less than I did prior to the pregnancy. With my second son, I gained about 25 pounds and it took me twice as long—about ten months—to lose the weight.

Breast-feeding increases your calorie needs and helps your uterus shrink quickly after childbirth. I breast-fed both of my kids for six months and was sure to keep my calorie intake up to maintain my milk supply. As long as your baby seems well fed and is growing well, you can safely and gradually cut your calorie intake to promote slow weight loss postpartum. Losing all the weight you gained after pregnancy and before subsequent pregnancies, can certainly help reduce your likelihood of becoming overweight or obese down the road.

Weight Gain Goals

It's a great idea to track your weight gain (your obstetrician will do this as well) to make sure you're consuming enough calories to support a healthy pregnancy. You can weigh yourself once a week or once a day—whatever helps you but doesn't make you crazy. Ever since I can remember, I have weighed myself daily. It helps keep me on track, and I believe it has helped keep off the 30 pounds I have lost over the years. The recommended rate and total amount of weight gain during pregnancy varies from person to person, and your own weight gain may fluctuate from week to week. Less than 5 pounds during the first trimester, and less than 1 pound a week (0.4 kilograms) is generally recommended (you can safely gain more weight if you're underweight prior to pregnancy or carrying twins, and you may aim for a slower rate of weight gain if you're overweight prior to pregnancy).

The following guidelines indicate how much weight to gain during pregnancy based on your prepregnancy body mass index (see appendix B to determine your BMI) and how many fetuses you're carrying.

Pregnancy Weight Gain: How Much Is Enough?	
Prepregnancy BMI (kg/m^3)	Weight Gain (pounds)
Low (<19.8)	28–40
Normal (19.8–26)	25–35
Overweight (>26–29)	15–25
Obese (>29)	15–20
Twin Gestation (any BMI)	35–45
Triplet gestation (any BMI)	50

Sources: Food and Nutrition Board, Institute of Medicine, Nutrition during Pregnancy. (Washington, DC: National Academy Press, 1990), and J.E. Brown and M. Carlson, "Nutrition and Multifetal Pregnancy," Journal of the American Dietetic Association 100 (2000): 343–48.

Calorie Goals

Although calorie needs do increase during pregnancy, "eating for two" is an overstatement. Calorie needs increase by about 300 calories—the amount in one slice of whole-wheat bread, 1 cup of skim milk, and a large banana—during the second and third trimesters to support fetal growth and women's changing bodies. How many calories you need while you are pregnant depends on how many calories you currently consume. If you're pregnant, try to meet your calorie needs by incorporating all the key food groups as recommended in chapter 10. If nausea strikes, or you have particular food aversions, it's okay to grab some crackers or guzzle down some ginger ale if that's all you can handle (cheese crackers and grape ginger ale were my antinausea snacks). If you feel hungrier during pregnancy (I know I did—both times) or crave sweet or snack-type foods that don't fit into any particular food category, I say go for it. Just keep portions small (about 100 calories) to satisfy your cravings without overdoing it.

Nutrient Goals

Pregnant women also need considerably more iron than ever before: 27 milligrams. If you are pregnant, be sure to consume foods that are high in heme iron (the kind found in animal foods) and/or non heme iron (the kind found in plant foods); pair these foods with those high in vitamin C to enhance iron absorption. (See appendix D for food sources of these key nutrients.)

Pregnant women need 600 micrograms of folic acid, a B vitamin that reduces the risk of neural tube defects that can lead to improper brain and spinal cord development in offspring. Luckily, many frequently consumed foods, such as ready-to-eat cereals and other grain products, are currently fortified with folic acid, which makes it much easier for women to incorporate more folic acid to meet their needs. See appendix D for other good food sources of folic acid.

Carbohydrate Goals

Carbohydrates provide the brain and red blood cells with much needed fuel that is the body's main energy source. They are also a good source of key nutrients such as B vitamins, folic acid, and fiber and can be found in abundance in vegetables, fruits, and grains, as well as in milk and beans. You can get ample carbohydrates by following the dietary pattern recommended in chapter 10. Whole grains, fruits, vegetables, and beans, in particular, provide a lot of fiber, which benefits your heart by lowering cholesterol levels, prevents constipation (which plagues many pregnant women), and promotes good overall gastrointestinal health. See appendix D for good sources of fiber.

Fat Goals

Recent studies show that getting enough DHA, an omega-3 fatty acid found in fish, during pregnancy and breast-feeding is critical for the cognitive development of offspring. Unfortunately, many pregnant women steer clear of fish altogether because of potential contamination with mercury and polychlorinated biphenyls (PCBs), compounds that can affect memory, behavior, and intellectual development in fetuses and infants. Pregnant women should avoid high-mercury fish such as shark, swordfish, king mackerel, and tilefish but can safely consume up to about 12 ounces of low-mercury fish including fresh or canned wild salmon, chunk light canned tuna, sardines, or herring each week to get adequate DHA and minimize any potential adverse effects. They may also want to have wild or Alaskan salmon instead of Atlantic or Icelandic farm-raised salmon that has higher levels of cancer-causing polychlorinated biphenyls (PCBs). Those who don't eat fish should speak with their doctor about supplemental DHA.

Protein Needs

Protein needs do increase during pregnancy, but because most people consume more protein than their bodies need to begin with, a woman who follows an appropriate dietary pattern based on her prepregnancy body weight (see chapter 10) will likely get enough to meet her needs.

Fluid Goals

Although you will make many more trips to the bathroom than usual, pregnancy is a time when fluid needs increase to support the increased blood volume of pregnancy and to avoid constipation. Be sure to choose water, seltzer, low-fat milk (1% or skim), 100% fruit juice, even a cup of coffee or tea, as well as plenty of fruits, vegetables, and broth-based or vegetable-based soups and cooked grains like oatmeal to meet your daily fluid needs. Drink regularly, and make sure to have extra fluid on hand if you sweat from exercise or it's hot outside.

Worldly Wise Goals

Avoid alcohol and stop smoking, keep caffeine at 300 mg per day or less, and avoid foods that can potentially contain bacteria that can harm you and your unborn fetus (see the resources at the end of the book for more on food safety).

Exercise Goals

Women who are physically active during pregnancy lower their risk for gestational diabetes (high blood sugar in pregnancy) by 50 percent compared with inactive women. Exercise also lowers the risk for preeclampsia (high blood pressure in pregnancy) by 40 percent. Despite these and other benefits, a recent study showed that only 1 in 6 pregnant women met current exercise guidelines (at least thirty minutes of moderate physical activity on most days of the week). Barring any medical complications, pregnant women can safely engage in moderate exercise. See appendix F for safe guidelines for exercise during pregnancy as well as ideas for how to incorporate more physical activity into your day.

Goals for Breast-Feeding

Breast-feeding appears to protect children from obesity. Studies show that the longer children are breast-fed, the less likely they are to become obese (the protective effect appears to be up to one year). Why is it protective? Breast milk appears to contain nutrients and bioactive substances that may favorably affect metabolism in infants. Also, the process of breast-feeding itself may help infants regulate their energy intake better and rely more on/be better in touch with their internal hunger cues because infants tend to stop sucking when they've had enough; bottle-fed babies may be encouraged to finish a bottle even though they've had enough (parents seldom want to see any milk left in a bottle).

Even though I was initially nervous about the idea of breast-feeding, I decided at least to try it, knowing what great health benefits it would provide for my son. Although the first month was indeed a challenge, after that it got much easier for me. I breast-fed my first son for six months and my second son (also a good feeder) for six months and one day (going one extra day with my second son was my attempt to make up for the inevitable neglect my second son would have to endure from me—I always heard how much less attention a second child gets). For me, breast-feeding was convenient (although it took me until I had my second son to breast-feed anywhere near another human being except my husband or my mother). It was also, for me, an amazing bonding experience. If you don't want to breast-feed, no one can force you to. Ultimately, you are the only one who can decide what's best for you and your child. If you do decide to try, hang on for at least a month. I started with a goal of one month, and then set a goal for three months, and then finally said six months would be my goal. If you can breast-feed up to a year, go for it (it does get easier with time); keep in mind that you won't need to nurse as frequently once you start to supplement your infant with table food (between four and six months). Also, older infants usually feed a lot faster than newborns. Working moms can breast-feed, too (I know several who did it in the morning and at night for up to a year after their three-month maternity leave; they pumped a few times during the day at work). Where there's a will there's a way.

If for whatever reason you cannot breast-feed or don't want to, you can still raise healthy and fit kids and be healthy and fit yourself. But breast-feeding can provide many wonderful health and other benefits to both you and your baby.

Figuring Out Yourself

Whether you are young, old, pregnant, never pregnant, an at-home mother or an entrepreneur or any combination of these, learning how to feel good about yourself—both inside and out—is a gift, not only for yourself but for your family. What husband constantly wants to answer the question "Honey, does this make me look fat?" or hear "My butt is so big." Talking negatively about your body, especially in front of your children, is useless and potentially destructive. Even if you don't feel great about every body part, your size and shape, or your physical appearance overall, turning the negative statements you think and say about yourself (and others as well) into positives will help you change how you think about yourself (and others). One of the ways I learned to accept my body a long time ago was to talk more positively about myself and focus on what I like about my looks and my body as opposed to focusing on what I wish I had. I didn't get thin legs, but I did get nice eyelashes and pretty hands. Sometimes writing down a few things you like about yourself in a journal can help. Surrounding yourself with people who support you and make you feel good about yourself, both inside and out, can also be invaluable.

So as you can see, being a woman can be tough. But gaining weight and losing our shape as we age is not inevitable, despite the obstacles and challenges that confront us. Being more mindful of what and how much we eat, how we use our bodies day to day, and the many negative things we say to ourselves and others about our weight, our bodies, and our appearance in general can help us on our quest to adopt a lifestyle that helps us look and feel better, manage our weight, achieve better overall health, and be a role model for healthy living to our children and others.

8

Men

When cave dwellers had to hunt to bring home food for their families, they were very physically fit and had no problems with excess weight. Their muscles were large and defined, their bellies were flat, and they were ready to run. Studies of the few isolated hunter-gatherer societies—the Nanamiut of Alaska, the Aborigines of Australia, and the Kung of Africa—that remained into the twentieth century found that modern maladies, such as heart disease, high cholesterol, obesity, and diabetes, were rare in these populations. There's no need for today's men to be on the hunt for their food. It's readily available to them with a quick phone call, a drive through a local fast-food outlet, or a stop at the cafeteria at work or convenience store around the corner from where they live. And although women are increasingly busy with their own work and family commitments, they often shop for, cook, or otherwise provide the men in their lives with food at mealtimes. For many of today's men, physical activity consists of cheering from a sofa while watching other men run around in some ball game and walking to their car or the train to ride to work.

The Reality for Men

No wonder that more and more men are becoming overweight or obese with no signs of a slowdown. Almost 71 percent of all men age twenty and above are currently considered obese or overweight. The average adult male weighs approximately 25 pounds more and is 1½ inches taller than he was in 1960 (191 pounds compared with 166 pounds). That's no surprise, given that men's daily calorie intake has risen by an estimated 7 percent, or 168 calories, over the last three decades, with most of these extra calories coming from carbohydrate-rich foods and beverages. Although obesity is less common in men than in women, a recent study found that men are catching up and increasingly become obese, as opposed to women who seem to be holding steady at 33 percent. Approximately 31 percent of men are now considered obese, compared with 28 percent just six years ago. Unlike in women, there is little difference in the rate of obesity among men with different racial or ethnic backgrounds.

More and more men are interested in losing weight, but they are reluctant to admit it. They describe women who diet as doing so for cosmetic reasons, whereas men prefer to think of themselves as dieting for legitimate reasons such as health. Going on a diet or joining a weight-loss support group to slim down is often perceived as a feminine pursuit, and men are typically less willing to undertake such efforts without support from their partners, other family members, or peers.

Although men are more active than women—almost half of them (about 48.2 percent) report at least thirty minutes a day of physical activity—22.2 percent report no leisure time physical activity. Men are often motivated to be buff and in good athletic shape; many are athletic as they grow up but engage less and less in sports as they enter the workforce and start a family. My husband, for example, was very active all through college but put on some weight once he moved to New York City, worked long hours (sometimes as much as one hundred hours a week), had little time to exercise, and relied heavily on take-out food for most of his meals. Like women, men lose lean muscle mass and gain body fat and weight as they get older, and more so if they eat more and move less because of work and family demands. Unfortunately, most men are apple shaped, and those extra calories often end up where they want them least—in their guts. Being thick around the middle, which plagues more men than women, greatly increases health risks (see the box "Apples versus Pears" on page 15).

Goals for Men

Following are some goals and tips to help men achieve and sustain a healthier body weight.

Calorie Goals

Because men tend to accumulate harmful belly fat, a realistic goal for many can be to prevent weight gain as they get older. If they want to lose weight, cutting portion sizes and watching liquid calories can certainly help trim their calorie intake. Because men tend to be taller and have more muscle mass and less body fat than women, their calorie needs are about 20 percent higher than those of women. In general, here are the daily calorie needs for weight maintenance in men who are sedentary:

Age	Calories per Day
21–40	2,400
41–60	2,200
61 and above	About 2,000

Nutrient Goals

Compared with women, men need more of many key nutrients, primarily because their calorie needs are higher. They need more protein, linolenic and alpha-linolenic acids, thiamin, riboflavin, niacin, vitamin K, choline, chromium, fluoride, and zinc, nutrients that can be obtained in the dietary pattern encouraged in chapter 10. Other key nutrients men need more than they tend to get include vitamin A, vitamin C, vitamin E, calcium, folate, magnesium, potassium, and fiber (see appendix D for key food sources of all these key nutrients.)

The Sleep Goal

Getting enough sleep is just as important for men as it is for women to help them function optimally and possibly prevent weight gain. Studies show that the less sleep men get, the more they tend to weigh. See the resources at the end of the book for more information on sleep.

The Battery Recharging Goal

Exercise can not only keep men energized but can help them preserve or build additional lean muscle mass to combat weight and fat gain that often occurs as men get older. Men tend to respond much more quickly to exercise than women do in terms of muscle gain and fat loss (much to the chagrin of women who tend to work so hard to achieve the same results). Perhaps having kids is a good incentive and excuse for men to take up sports or do activities with their kids that they haven't done since their own childhood, such as shooting baskets, throwing a football, or playing baseball in the backyard. These are some easy ways families can increase the fitness of all members. For tips and ideas for how to get started, see chapter 3.

One Step at a Time

With just a little effort, men can achieve a healthier body weight. Because they require more calories than women, they don't need to make as many calorie cuts to reduce their overall intake and subsequently lose weight. Also, because they often have a lot of muscle mass to begin with, adding some extra weight training and cardiovascular exercise increases their calorie burn even more. Just a few weeks of subtle calorie cuts and a few short weight-training and cardiovascular exercise sessions can lead to noticeable results, which can be a real motivator for men. This can help them not only look and feel stronger and more fit but can help them maintain a healthy body weight and potentially reduce their risks down the road for chronic diseases such as heart disease, type 2 diabetes, and cancer.

9

Seniors

As you get older, it gets tougher to maintain a healthy body weight. That's because you're likely less active than you used to be, which can lead you to lose some muscle mass and accumulate more fat mass (especially in the abdominal area). You also need fewer calories to maintain your weight with each passing decade. Calorie needs drop by about 2 or 3 percent, which equals about 40 to 60 calories a day (the equivalent of a cookie) for most people. As you get older and take in fewer calories, your body responds by burning fewer calories. Changing hormones also affect body weight as you get older and can lead to increases in body fat, decreases in lean muscle mass, and other effects on appetite and energy balance that contribute to weight gain. Managing a healthful body weight can also be a challenge if you're on certain medications, including steroids.

The Reality for Seniors

Although older adults are more likely to be obese than their younger counterparts, those over the age of eighty were obese at a similar rate to twenty- to thirty-nine-year-olds. In addition to obesity, however, older people may also be plagued by another weight problem: underweight. Weight loss or weight gain, especially when you're older, may be red flags for health problems. According to the National Health and Nutrition Examination Survey (NHANES), as many as 16 percent of Americans over the age of sixty-five consume less than 1,000 calories a day, which puts them at severe risk of malnutrition.

If you live alone, have limited interaction with others, have to fend for yourself, and do all your own food shopping and prepare all your own meals, it may be easy to skip meals or eat less than you need. If you're on medications that affect your sense of taste, or if you have any physical limitations that make it tough for you to move around, your food intake and physical activity may decrease.

But it's never too late (and no one is ever too old) to make changes in the way you eat and move your body to better manage your weight, improve your strength and feelings of well-being, and enhance your health and overall quality of life. There are, of course, some challenges to making changes in how you eat and how you move. For one, you're likely quite set in your ways (I know my parents are). Most people don't like to change, so even though you'd like to weigh less or feel more energetic, wanting to make changes and actually taking steps to do so are two different things. Or perhaps you're caring for an older parent yourself, or a spouse, or your own children or grandchildren. This may leave you little time to take care of yourself and focus on your own unique needs. Perhaps you have a medical condition (or more than one) that affects how you eat or limits your ability to exercise and be physically fit. Depression and taking medications for medical conditions can also make good eating and fitness habits a real challenge unless you make a real effort to change. See the resources for older adults at the end of the book.

Goals for Seniors

Following are some calorie and nutrient goals, as well as physical activity goals, that you can work toward achieving, no matter what your age. Your body and mind will certainly benefit when you take steps to improve your current food and fitness habits.

Calorie Goals

Although many older people are still concerned about the number on the scale and their appearance, preventing or managing diet-related diseases is often incentive enough to watch calorie intake. Here is an estimate of calorie needs, based on a sedentary level of daily physical activity, for older adults who want to manage their weight:

	Age	Calories per Day
Women	51 and above	1,600
Men	51–60	2,200
	61 and above	2,000

See chapter 10 to find a dietary pattern based on your suggested calorie level.

Nutrient Goals

Older adults, both women and men, need more calcium than they did when they were younger, with the exception of adolescence when calcium needs are highest (about 1,300 mg per day). When women around the age of fifty go through menopause, their estrogen levels decline, which significantly increases the breakdown of bone that makes women especially susceptible to bone fractures. And although genetics play a large part in how much bone women can build over their lifetime, diet (getting enough calcium) and incorporating weight training into their routine can help women preserve bone as they get older. (See appendix D and chapter 3.)

Vitamin D is another key nutrient older people need because it increases calcium absorption and reduces the risk for bone loss; the needs for vitamin D double to 10 micrograms (or 400 International Units, or IU) for both women and men during their fifties and sixties and triple to 15 micrograms per day (or 600 IU) when they reach their seventies. Older people need to make sure to get adequate vitamin D from a combination of sunlight (vitamin D is made when the skin is exposed to sunlight), food, and/or supplements. (See appendix D for food sources of vitamin D.)

Some experts recommend as much as 1,000 IU of vitamin D each day for adults because good quality sunlight is not always available, especially during the winter months in some parts of the country, and because few older people get vitamin D from food sources. Currently, less than 10 percent of older adults (fifty-one to seventy years old) and only about 2 percent of those over age seventy consume adequate vitamin D from food sources alone. Because of this, older people should discuss vitamin D supplementation with a physician, especially if they don't consume vitamin D–rich foods often.

Some B vitamins are also increasingly important for older people. Vitamin B_{12} helps form red blood cells and maintain a healthy nervous system. Older people don't need more vitamin B_{12}, but an estimated 10 to 30 percent of those over the age of fifty may have a reduced ability to absorb it according to a recent report by the Dietary Guidelines for Americans Advisory Committee. People over age fifty are advised to consume vitamin B_{12} in its crystalline form (for example, in food or supplements) and may want to discuss vitamin B_{12} supplementation with a physician. People above the age of fifty-one also need extra vitamin B_6, which is involved in many body functions including protein metabolism. See appendix D for a list of foods rich in vitamin B_6.

Physical Activity Goals

According to the Centers for Disease Control, only 37 percent of Americans older than age sixty-five get the recommended amount of physical activity—thirty minutes of moderate exercise—on most, if not all, days. Another 35 percent of people in this age group do not meet this minimum amount of exercise, and 28 percent get no exercise. Older people with chronic health problems including heart disease, hypertension, diabetes, osteoporosis, asthma, or obesity; those who do not currently exercise; and anyone who plans to begin vigorous physical activity should play it safe and consult with their doctors before they begin any exercise program. Depending on where you're starting from, it's best to start slowly. You can incorporate weight training, cardiovascular exercise, and some stretching, but make sure to have some guidance from a qualified fitness professional (see the resources at the end of the book). Any exercise program you begin should be gradual, realistic, and take into account your personal exercise, medical, and weight history, and it must be based on your needs, abilities, and personal preferences. See chapter 3 for more tips to help you fit in fitness.

Getting older does not mean you can't achieve and maintain a healthier body weight. It also doesn't mean you can't improve your body composition to build muscle mass and preserve your metabolism. You may have to work a little harder than when you were younger, but it can be done with just a little bit of effort. Getting support from friends who want to achieve similar goals or from younger family members is a great way to stay motivated and help you maintain more healthful food and fitness habits long term.

part three

The Family Action Plan

10

The Ultimate Family Food Guide

Here's where all the fun truly begins! In this chapter, you and your family will learn not only what you *can* eat but how to balance out your food choices and in proper proportions to help you meet your individual calorie and nutrient needs and achieve and maintain a healthier body weight. You'll see that you won't have to give up any of your favorite foods but will be guided toward choosing wholesome, nutrient-dense foods to help you get started on your way toward healthier eating habits. I've created the Ultimate Family Food Guide: a one-stop reference that employs the principles of the *Dietary Guidelines for Americans 2005* for what and how much you and your family can aim for on any given day, based on your individual age and gender. (See the table on page 96.)

The calorie recommendations in this guide (which range from 900 calories for one-year-olds up to 2,600 calories for nineteen- to twenty-year-old men) are approximations of what you and individual family members need each day to achieve and maintain healthier body weights. If you already do regular moderate or vigorous physical activity on most days of the week (for example, if you go the gym several days a week or play competitive team sports), you may need more calories to maintain your current body weight. If weight loss is your goal, the recommended calorie levels are a good place to start to help you lose weight slowly and gradually. As you can see, calorie needs

The Ultimate Family Food Guide

Males	Females	Calories per Day	Fruits (cups)	Vegetables (cups)	Grains (1-ounce equivalents)	Meat and Beans (1-ounce equivalents)	Milk, Yogurt, Cheese (1-cup equivalents)	Oils (teaspoons)	Extra Calories
1	1	900	1	¾	2	1½	2	1	100
2–3	2–3	1,000	1	1	3	2	2	3	150
4–5	4–7	1,200	1	1½	4	3	2	3½	150
6–8	8–10	1,400	1½	1½	5	4	2	3½	150
9–10	11–13, 51+	1,600	1½	2	5	5	3	5	200
11–12	14–18, 26–50	1,800	1½	2½	6	5	3	5	200
13–14, 61+	19–25	2,000	2	2½	6	5½	3	6	250
15, 41–60		2,200	2	3	7	6	3	6	300
16–18, 21–40		2,400	2	3	8	6½	3	7	350
19–20		2,600	2	3½	9	6½	3	7	400

vary widely, so most individuals in your family will have a unique meal pattern. Keep the Ultimate Family Food Guide on your refrigerator or a bulletin board in your kitchen as a quick reminder of your daily food intake goals.

To estimate your individual calorie needs, see the columns labeled "females" and "males" on the left-hand side of the chart on page 96. Select your gender, and then go down the column to find your age. Once you find your age, move your finger across that row to find your estimated calorie needs, followed by the minimum number of portions of all the different food groups—fruits, vegetables, grains, meat and beans, milk/yogurt/cheese, and oils—to aim for each day. In the last column, you'll find extra calories. These are included in the calorie estimates and range from 150 to 400 calories based on your recommended calorie level. These extras can be used on any foods or beverages you choose, including sugary treats or wine or you can simply use them to have extra helpings of any items within the various food categories.

Once you've figured out your personal meal pattern, it's time to eat! But before you dive in, first learn the wide range of foods from which you and your family members can choose and how to fit those foods into your individual dietary patterns. Following are more thorough descriptions of the various food categories illustrated in the Ultimate Family Food Guide. Anyone in your family older than age one can use this guide (as well as the family meal plans and recipes in chapters 14 and 15) as a template for eating in a way that supports good overall health and healthy weight management. (See page 55 for a sample menu and page 54 for "Top Tips for Feeding Your Under-Twos.")

Fill Up on Fruits

As part of a nutrient-dense diet, fruit is a superstar. It is loaded with key nutrients, including vitamin A, vitamin C, potassium, and antioxidants, substances that can help prevent type 2 diabetes, heart disease, cancer, and other conditions. Fruit can also be a useful ally in your weight management efforts because it's naturally high in water content as well as in fiber and can therefore fill you up on relatively few calories. Fruit is easily accessible and portable, and it makes a great on-the-go snack. It can also be easily used to perk up meals or snacks with some natural sweetness (see page 98 for tips to help you and your family consume more fruit).

How Much to Aim for Each Day

Between 1 and 2 cups of fruit are recommended for family members based on their estimated calorie level. See the table on page 96 to determine how many cups of fruit to aim for each day.

What Counts as a Fruit?

Any fresh, frozen, canned, or dried fruit, or 100% fruit juice can count toward meeting your daily quota for fruit intake. Emphasize fruit products made without added sugar. In general, here's what counts as ½ cup of fruit (see appendix G to find specific foods in this category):

- ½ cup cut-up raw or cooked or frozen fruit
- 1 medium fruit (for example, a small banana, orange, or peach)
- ½ cup 100% fruit juice (for example, apple juice, cranberry juice, or orange juice)

Here are some tips to encourage your family to consume more fruit at meals and snacks:

- Keep a clear bowl filled with fresh fruit such as bananas, pears, apples, and oranges on your kitchen counter and restock every few days.
- Top whole-grain or bran cereal with sliced bananas, strawberries, peaches, or apricots.
- Add applesauce, bananas, or blueberries to whole-grain pancake, waffle, or muffin mix.
- Use fresh berries, crushed pineapple, or dried fruit to top low-fat yogurt.
- Keep a see-through container filled with cut-up fresh fruit in the refrigerator for easy access.

Suggested Daily Amount of Fruit	
Calorie Level	Amount (in Cups)
900–1,200	1
1,400–1,800	1½
2,000–2,600	2

- Dip melon balls or fresh fruit slices into low-fat yogurt or mix with low-fat cottage cheese.
- Add grapes, apple slices, orange sections, or dried fruit to salad greens.
- Make a sandwich with whole-grain bread, peanut butter, and banana or apple slices.
- Dip apple slices into peanut butter or salsa.
- Freeze grapes for a cold snack or fill ice cube trays with 100% fruit juice (such as orange juice) and toothpicks to make ice pops.
- Add fresh fruit slices to plain water or seltzer.
- Bake an apple and top it with cinnamon for dessert or a quick midday snack.
- Keep natural applesauce or canned fruit cups without added sugar for a portable on-the-go snack.
- Make fruit kebobs with fresh chunks of pineapple and melon, or add to chicken, steak, or fish kebobs at your next barbecue.

Don't Forget Your Vegetables

Vegetables are great sources of vitamins A and C, potassium, and iron, not to mention antioxidants (disease-fighting substances). They provide little fat, and because they are high in fiber and loaded with water, they are very filling. As an added bonus, most vegetables are low in calories, which makes them great to consume especially when you're watching your weight.

How Much to Aim for Each Day

Between ¾ and 3½ cups of vegetables are recommended for family members based on their estimated calorie level. See the table on page 100 to determine how many cups of vegetables to aim for each day.

What Counts as a Vegetable?

All fresh, frozen, and canned vegetables and vegetable juices that are made or prepared without any added sugars or fats count toward helping you meet your daily quota for vegetables. Here's what counts as ½ cup of vegetables (see appendix G to find specific foods in this category):

Suggested Daily Amount of Vegetables	
Calorie Level	Amount (in Cups)
900	¾
1,000	1
1,200–1,400	1½
1,600	2
1,800–2,000	2½
2,200–2,400	3
2,600	3½

- ½ cup cut-up raw or cooked vegetables (including starchy vegetables like potatoes)
- ½ cup vegetable juice
- 1 cup leafy salad greens
- ¼ cup legumes or soybean products (including dry beans and peas such as pinto beans, kidney beans, lentils, chickpeas, and tofu)

Legumes and soybean products may be counted as vegetables or meat and beans (see page 105); if you eat large amounts of these foods (for example, if you follow a vegan or vegetarian diet), be sure to keep an eye on how much you consume so as not to exceed your recommended calorie level.

Aim for a Rainbow of Nutrients

Most Americans, especially kids, are not consuming enough vegetables. Because different vegetables provide different combinations of key nutrients, it's important for everyone to include a variety of vegetables to ensure adequate nutrient intake. Each week, be sure to include several portions of these brightly colored vegetables:

- **Dark green vegetables** such as asparagus, broccoli, brussels sprouts, romaine and other leafy greens, spinach, and zucchini
- **Orange and deep-yellow vegetables** such as butternut squash, carrots, corn, summer squash, sweet potatoes, winter squash, and pumpkin
- **Legumes** such as lentils, white kidney beans, sugar snap peas, tofu, and tempeh

Following are some tips to encourage your family to incorporate more vegetables at meals and snacks:

- Stock up on a variety of vegetables—canned and frozen (with no salt or fat added) as well as fresh—to provide a range of options as well as a variety of tastes and textures.
- Keep washed ready-to-eat vegetables such as celery stalks, baby carrots, cucumber slices, and grape tomatoes in a clear bowl in the refrigerator for easy access; eat alone or dip in low-fat salad dressing or yogurt dip for a quick snack.
- Offer non-starchy vegetables at meals; round them out with either a starchy vegetable such as potatoes or corn, or a grain.
- Add chopped asparagus, mushrooms, onions, tomatoes, or red, green, or yellow peppers in any combination to scrambled eggs or omelets.
- Add chopped tomato to a toasted whole-grain English muffin and top with shredded mozzarella or cheddar cheese.
- Add broccoli florets to macaroni and cheese.
- Add unsalted canned corn, peas, and carrots to classic macaroni and cheese or pasta with tomato sauce for some added taste and texture.
- Top cooked vegetables with grated parmesan cheese or some melted cheddar cheese.
- Top a baked potato with broccoli florets or chopped asparagus lightly sauteed in olive oil.
- Use celery sticks as a base for natural peanut or almond butter topped with raisins or other dried fruit.
- Add sweet potatoes to a small amount of whole-grain pancake mix for a tasty breakfast or dinner side dish.
- Have a vegetable or bean-based soup as a starter for lunch or dinner.
- Add a few slices of tomato, romaine, or raw spinach to sandwiches.
- Top a slice of crusty bread with grilled vegetables such as eggplant, red or green peppers, or zucchini drizzled with vinaigrette.
- Have a large colorful salad with a mix of crunchy vegetables such as broccoli and carrots, and beans such as chickpeas.
- Make a vegetable stir-fry, and use it to top pasta, baked skinless chicken, or fish.

- Make a baked ziti or lasagna dish with crushed fresh or low-sodium canned tomatoes, yellow peppers, and other colorful vegetables.

- Instead of your usual potato, bake squash and serve in cubes alongside poultry, fish, or a lean meat dish.

- Add shredded carrots, chopped fresh tomatoes, onions, or zucchini to meatball and meatloaf recipes.

- Make pizza with your kids: spread tomato sauce on pizza dough and add any combination of chopped or sliced vegetables such as mushrooms, green peppers, onions, and broccoli; sprinkle with mozzarella or grated parmesan cheese; bake and serve.

- Use puréed, cooked vegetables such as potatoes or squash as a thickener for soups and stews.

- Grill zucchini, carrots, and eggplant slices at your next barbecue.

- Add puréed carrots, zucchini, or pumpkin to muffin mixes.

- Dip raw vegetable slices into hummus for a protein-packed snack.

Go for Glorious Grains

Grains provide the body with many key nutrients. First and foremost, they provide carbohydrates, the key fuel for the brain and the entire central nervous system. Grains are also important vehicles for dietary fiber, B vitamins such as folate, thiamin, riboflavin, and niacin, and minerals including iron, magnesium, and selenium. The two main categories of grains are whole grains and refined grains. Whole grains are intact, which means they include the entire grain kernel: the bran (the outer layer that contains fiber), the germ (the nutrient-rich inner part), and the endosperm (the middle layer). Refined grains are milled, a process that removes the bran and germ components. The grains are stripped of fiber, iron, and many B vitamins. Many refined grains are enriched, however, which means that iron and many B vitamins are added back after processing. Although all grains, whole or refined, can be included in a healthful diet, it's best to emphasize whole grains because they tend to be higher in fiber (which fills you up and can aid weight management) and help prevent heart disease, stroke, type 2 diabetes, and some cancers.

How Much to Aim for Each Day

A wide range or grains—between 2 and 9 1-ounce equivalents—is recommended for family members based on their estimated calorie levels. The *Dietary Guidelines for Americans 2005* encourage people to consume at least half of their total allotment of grains from whole grains; for example, if you consume 1,800 calories a day, aim for at least three out of your six grain servings in total to come from whole grains. See the table on this page to determine how many 1-ounce equivalents of grains to aim for each day.

What Counts as a Grain?

The following count as a 1-ounce equivalent of grains (see appendix G to find more foods in this category):

Whole grains:
- 1 cup ready-to-eat whole-grain cereal flakes
- ½ cup cooked oatmeal
- 1 ounce (usually 1 slice) whole-wheat and rye breads
- 1 ounce dry or ½ cup cooked brown rice
- 1 ounce dry or ½ cup cooked whole-wheat pasta
- 1 ounce whole-wheat crackers (approximately three to five crackers)

Suggested Daily Amounts of Grains	
Calorie Level	Amount (in 1-ounce equivalents)
900	2
1,000	3
1,200	4
1,400–1,600	5
1,800–2,000	6
2,200	7
2,400	8
2,600	9

Refined grains:
- 1 slice white bread
- 1 cup cereal flakes made with enriched grains
- 1 ounce crackers made with enriched grains
- 1 ounce dry or ½ cup cooked white rice
- 1 ounce dry or ½ cup cooked pasta

Because most Americans fall short on whole grains and average only about one 1-ounce equivalent each day, here are some tips to fill the whole-grain void in your family meals:

- Start your day with whole-grain, high-fiber cereal with low-fat milk and fresh fruit slices; if you or your kids currently consume a sugary cereal, you can mix ½ cup of that cereal with a healthier one to ease the transition.
- Use a crunchy whole-grain, high-fiber cereal as a topping for low-fat yogurt.
- Toast whole-wheat bread or a whole-wheat English muffin or pita and serve with melted low-fat cheese and scrambled egg whites.
- Sprinkle wheat germ into low-fat yogurt, salads, or pancake or waffle mix for a fiber boost.
- When baking muffins, cakes, or cookies, use oat or whole-wheat flour to replace at least a quarter or half of the white flour in the recipe.
- Offer different shaped whole-wheat pasta (for example, fusilli, penne, or macaroni) to make macaroni and cheese; you'd be surprised that if you offer this, especially at a young age, your kids will devour it. I know mine do!
- Offer brown rice or wild rice more often than white; throw in some lightly sautéed mixed vegetables to add some extra flavor.
- Add whole grains such as barley to homemade vegetable soups or bulgur wheat to stir-fries or casseroles.
- Toast and chop whole-wheat bread or use crushed whole-grain flaky cereals to make breadcrumbs to use as a coating for chicken cutlets, fish sticks, or vegetables such as onions or eggplant; bake and serve.
- Top whole-grain crackers with natural peanut butter, almond butter, soy butter, or hummus for a quick and easy treat packed with protein.

- Munch on air-popped or canola-oil popped popcorn instead of your usual chips.
- Use whole-wheat flour tortillas to make cheese, bean, chicken, or steak quesadillas or fajitas.
- Experiment with less common grains including amaranth, millet, sorghum, triticale, and quinoa.

Add Some Lean Meats and Beans

Lean meats and beans provide an array of vitamins including niacin, vitamin B_6, and vitamin E as well as the mineral zinc. Dry beans and peas (which can also count as vegetables) also provide a good amount of fiber. Incorporating some foods from the meat and beans category at meals and snacks is a great vehicle for protein, a key nutrient needed not only for growth and repair of all body tissues but to help fill you up at meals and prevent rapid swings in blood sugar levels between meals that can lead to excessive hunger (and subsequently to overeating). However, because many foods in this category are high in calories, and many options, especially meat and poultry choices, may contain significant amounts of total fat, saturated fat, and cholesterol depending on their cuts and how they're prepared, keep portions small and choose foods from the meat and beans category wisely (see chapter 12 for shopping tips). Nevertheless, to manage a healthy body weight, consume some good protein sources each time you eat; the meat and beans food category can provide many wonderful options.

How Much to Aim for Each Day

Between 1½ and 6½ 1-ounce equivalents of meat and beans are recommended for family members based on their estimated calorie level. See the table on page 106 to determine how many 1-ounce equivalents of meat and beans to aim for each day.

What Foods Are Included in the Meat and Beans Category?

Meat, poultry, fish, dry beans and peas, eggs, nuts, seeds, and soy foods in their most lean and low-fat form (for example, skinless white meat chicken, sirloin steak, or low-fat soy milk) are included in the meat and

Suggested Daily Amounts of Meat and Beans	
Calorie Level	Amount (in 1-ounce equivalents)
900	1½
1,000	2
1,200	3
1,400	4
1,600–1,800	5
2,000	5½
2,200	6
2,400–2,600	6½

beans category. The following count as a 1-ounce equivalent (see appendix G to find more foods in this category):

- 1 ounce fish including cod, haddock, catfish
- 1 ounce lean poultry (skinless, white meat)
- 1 ounce lean meat
- ¼ cup cooked dry beans
- ¼ cup tofu
- 1 tablespoon peanut butter
- ½ ounce nuts or seeds
- 1 egg

Peanut butter, nuts, and seeds naturally contain oils. To help you achieve your nutrient needs without exceeding your calorie allotment, count 1 tablespoon of peanut butter (or another nut butter) or ½ ounce of nuts and seeds as a 1-ounce equivalent of meat and beans plus 1 teaspoon of oil.

Following are some tips for how you and your family can incorporate more nutrient-dense meat and bean options into your meals:

- Sprinkle shaved nuts or seeds onto whole-grain cereal or low-fat yogurt.
- Add a sliced hard-boiled egg to a salad for a boost of protein and flavor.
- Add natural peanut butter, almond butter, or soy butter to whole-grain toast, whole-wheat crackers, or celery stalks.
- Have a vegetable burger on a whole-grain bun.

EZ Quick Tip: Get Healthy with Fish

Fish and shellfish can be a healthful part of everyone's diet because they are not only great sources of protein but they are low in saturated fat and loaded with essential nutrients. Fish also provides healthful omega-3 fats, polyunsaturated fats that can play a role in heart health as well as neurological development of offspring. Fish is also relatively low in calories, and therefore replacing higher fat meats and poultry with fish a few times a week can help you and your family curb your calorie intake. Because many people, especially women of childbearing age, worry about mercury and other contaminants in fish, they avoid fish completely or simply don't consume enough (nor do their family members, including their children) to derive the heart-healthy and other benefits fish provides. Although almost all fish and shellfish do contain traces of mercury, this poses little risk for most people. The Food and Drug Administration and the Environmental Protection Agency advise women who may become pregnant, women who are pregnant or nursing, and young children to do the following:

- Avoid the following fish that contain high levels of mercury: shark, swordfish, tilefish, or king mackerel.

- Consume a variety of low-mercury fish (up to 12 ounces per week); some popular low-mercury fish include shrimp, canned light tuna, salmon, pollock, and catfish. If you choose albacore (white) tuna (canned or fresh), have no more than 6 ounces of it each week because it contains more mercury than canned light tuna.

- If you eat locally caught fish but have no information about its mercury content, it's prudent to limit your weekly intake to 6 ounces of that fish.

- Add walnuts, pecans, sunflower seeds, or chickpeas to salads.
- Mix a can of light tuna in water (drained) or grilled chicken strips to salad greens.
- Add kidney or pinto beans to a chili dish.
- Make a bean quesadilla or fajita with lentils or black beans and melted low-fat cheddar cheese.
- Add tofu with added calcium to stir fries and salads.
- Add toasted pine nuts to vegetable side dishes like green beans or spinach.
- Make a trail mix with nuts, dried fruit, and crunchy whole-grain cereal.

- Add chopped nuts to muffin and cookie recipes.
- Spread hummus on a toasted whole-wheat pita or on whole-grain crackers.
- Use lean meats such as skinless white meat chicken or turkey or round or loin cuts of beef as an addition to a vegetable-heavy stir-fry.
- Serve canned sardines on whole-grain toast or crackers to provide healthful omega-3 fats.

Go for Milk, Yogurt, and Cheese

Milk and milk products are important vehicles for key nutrients such as calcium, potassium, vitamin D, and protein. Including milk and milk products that are low in fat can help lower the risk for low bone mass in people of all ages. Some emerging research also suggests that including low-fat dairy foods as part of a reduced-calorie diet and exercise program can enhance weight loss and fat loss (specifically from the abdominal area). This research is fascinating but far from conclusive, but the bounty of nutrients found in milk, yogurt, and cheese and their great taste make this food group a great addition to a balanced, healthful diet.

How Much to Aim for Each Day

Two to three 1-cup equivalents of milk are recommended each day for all family members age one and older depending on their initial calorie levels. Children between the ages of one and two should be given whole milk; those above the age of two can make a gradual transition to low-fat milks and milk products until they regularly consume 1% or skim milk and other low-fat dairy foods. To limit calories and saturated fat, adults can aim to have mostly low-fat milk, yogurt, cheese, and other milk products. See the following table to determine how many 1-cup equivalents of milk to aim for each day.

| Suggested Daily Amounts of Milk ||
Calorie Level	Amount (in 1-cup equivalents)
900–1,400	2
1,600–2,600	3

The following count as a 1-cup equivalent of milk (see appendix G to find more foods in this category):

- 1 cup skim milk
- 1 cup nonfat yogurt
- 1½ ounces natural cheese
- 2 ounces processed cheese

With the exception of skim milk, all choices in the milk, yogurt, and cheese category provide extra calories. The table on this page lists some foods that count as a 1-cup equivalent of milk as well as extra calories. (See page 113.)

Following are some tips to help you and your family incorporate more low-fat or nonfat milk, yogurt, cheese, or other milk products into your meals and snacks:

- If you usually drink whole milk, switch gradually to fat-free milk to lower your saturated fat and calorie intake; try reduced fat (2%), then low-fat (1%), and finally fat-free (skim) milk.
- Serve skim or 1% milk with a straw.
- Add skim or 1% milk to your morning cereal.

Foods That Count as a 1-Cup Equivalent of Milk Plus Extra Calories*		
Amount	Approximate Calories	Count As
1 cup 1% milk	100	1 milk plus 20 extra calories
1 cup 2% milk	125	1 milk plus 40 extra calories
1 cup low-fat chocolate milk	160	1 milk plus 75 extra calories
1 cup whole milk	145	1 milk plus 65 extra calories
1 cup nonfat plain yogurt	100	1 milk plus 20 extra calories
1 cup low-fat plain yogurt	140	1 milk plus 60 extra calories
1 cup fruit-flavored low-fat yogurt	240–250	1 milk plus 110–115 extra calories
1½ ounces natural cheddar cheese	170	1 milk plus 90 extra calories
2 ounces processed American cheese	170	1 milk plus 90 extra calories

*Children between ages one and two do not need to count one cup of whole milk as one cup of milk plus 65 extra calories; these extra calories are allotted in their meal plan as shown in chapter 5.

- Add skim or 1% milk (instead of cream or higher-fat milks) to your coffee, or ask that your cappuccinos or lattes be made with skim or 1% milk.

- Top low-fat yogurt with fruit slices, dried fruit, or crunchy whole-grain cereal.

- Use skim or 1% milk to make oatmeal or other hot cereals, pancakes, or waffles.

- Mix low-fat or nonfat plain yogurt with fresh fruit chunks to make a smoothie, or add crunchy whole-grain cereal to make a breakfast parfait.

- Make whole-grain yogurt muffins with low-fat vanilla yogurt.

- Mix low-fat or nonfat plain yogurt with low-sodium onion broth or raw gelatin to make a quick dip for fruit chunks or vegetable strips.

- Use skim or 1% milk to make chocolate, vanilla, or butterscotch pudding.

- Use low-fat shredded cheese to top soups, casseroles, egg dishes, salads, or cooked vegetables.

- Top a baked potato with nonfat or low-fat plain yogurt.

- If after several failed efforts your kids still refuse to get enough milk into their diets, you can offer flavored low-fat or nonfat yogurt or chocolate milk; just be aware that often these contain more calories and sugar, which count as extra calories (see page 113 for a more complete explanation of extra calories).

- Keep reduced-fat string cheese on hand as a high-protein, grab-and-go snack.

If you or any family members avoid milk because of lactose intolerance, you can choose lactose-free milks and cheeses or take lactase supplements to help you better digest dairy foods. If you don't consume milk or other dairy products because of lactose intolerance, a milk allergy, or for taste reasons, you will need to make an extra effort to get enough calcium to meet your needs. You can find calcium in nondairy sources including fish, green vegetables, soy foods, beans, and fortified foods (such as ready-to-eat cereals and 100% fruit juices). See appendix D for a more specific list of nondairy calcium-rich foods and beverages.

Focus on Oils

Oils are fats that are liquid at room temperature. They come from plant sources (they naturally occur in nuts, seeds, avocado, and olives) as well as from fish. Many plant sources of oils, vegetable and nut oils, provide good amounts of vitamin E as well as healthful monounsaturated and polyunsaturated fats (including essential fats, those we need to get from our diets because our bodies can't make them). They are also cholesterol free. Oils and oily plant foods add a lot of flavor and texture to foods, but because they're a concentrated source of calories—they contain about 45 calories per teaspoon—we need to use small amounts when we cook with them or otherwise add them to foods.

What Foods Count as Oils?

Any healthful vegetable or nut oils that you add to food while cooking or at the table, or processed foods made with such oils (such as trans fat–free margarines, salad dressings, and mayonnaise) count as oils. Some fruits, including avocados and olives, naturally contain oils and are counted as oils. Nuts, nut butters, and seeds, however, which naturally contain oils, can be counted as both meat and beans (because of their high protein content; see the meat and beans food category on page 105) as well as oils; each ½ ounce of nuts or seeds, or tablespoon of peanut butter counts as a 1-ounce equivalent of meat and beans plus 1 teaspoon of oil.

How Much to Aim for Each Day

Up to 7 teaspoons of oil are recommended each day for all family members depending on their initial calorie levels. See the table one page 112 to see how many teaspoons of oil to aim for each day.

The following count as 1 teaspoon of oil (see appendix G to find more foods in this category):

- 1 teaspoon of:
  - canola oil
  - corn oil
  - cottonseed oil
  - olive oil

safflower oil

soybean oil

sunflower oil

walnut oil

sesame oil

mayonnaise (full fat)

- 1 tablespoon of:

    light or low-fat mayonnaise

    most salad dressings

- 2 tablespoons light salad dressing
- ⅓ cup avocado, sliced
- 15 small black olives, pitted
- 10 large black olives, pitted
- 7 green olives (queen size)
- 12 stuffed green olives
- ½ ounce nuts or nut butters (also count as 1-ounce equivalent of meat and beans)

Salad dressings and olives, especially, contain significant amounts of sodium (one olive alone has anywhere between 27 and 110 milligrams of sodium), so try to keep the amounts of these foods you consume small; this is particularly important if you have hypertension or are salt sensitive.

Unfortunately, most people consume too many oils (even healthful ones) to begin with. The best way to reduce your oil consumption is to limit how often and how much you add to foods. Here are some quick

Suggested Daily Amounts of Oil	
Calorie Level	Amount (in teaspoons)
900	1
1,000	3
1,200–1,400	3½
1,600–1,800	5
2,000–2,200	6
2,400–2,600	7

and simple ways you and your family can curb your intake without sacrificing taste:

- When you make salads, toss them well and serve without the dressing; keep the salad dressing on the side, and use your fork to dip into it with each bite.
- Replace 1 teaspoon of full-fat mayonnaise with 1 tablespoon of low-fat mayonnaise in your tuna or chicken salad recipe. If you prefer regular mayonnaise to the low-fat version, use only a small amount and add spices and seasonings, crunchy vegetables (such as carrots, celery, or peppers), fruit (chopped seedless red grapes), or mustard or balsamic vinegar to add more taste and texture.
- Use nonstick cooking spray instead of oil to prepare egg dishes (omelets or scrambled eggs), pancakes, or baked dishes (even baked French fries) without sacrificing flavor.
- Instead of mayonnaise on sandwiches, you can use mustard or balsamic vinegar to add flavor with few calories.
- When you bake, substitute half the amount of oil with natural applesauce to cut calories and fat.
- If you coat fish, chicken, or vegetables with breading to make them more tasty for your family, bake them instead of frying to prevent the food from mopping up excess oil.
- Use shredded low-fat cheese or grated parmesan cheese instead of oil on potatoes or cooked vegetables.
- Grill, bake, broil, or roast instead of frying; this will save you both calories and fat; use low-fat plain yogurt, salsa, chutney, mustard, balsamic vinegar, lemon juice, garlic, curry powder, parsley, rosemary, dill, and other flavorings to top fish, poultry, and meats.

Count Those Extra Calories

The Ultimate Family Food Guide (see page 96) allows for some extra calories. These calories are part of the estimated calorie amounts recommended for each family member based on their age and gender, and they represent calories beyond those obtained from the food categories just discussed. Extra calories are essentially calories that can be used any way you wish, depending on your individual food preferences. Each family member above the age of one is allotted anywhere between

100 and 400 calories each day. Extra calories can be used for any foods or beverages you choose, including sugary treats or wine, or you can simply use these extra calories for extra helpings of any items within the various food categories. If you incorporate the most healthful foods and beverages from each food group (that is, you choose the lowest fat, lowest sugar options within each category), you and your family can incorporate extra calories and still have healthful, nutrient-dense, and balanced diets that support your weight management goals.

The table on this page shows an approximation of how many extra calories you and your family can afford based on individual calorie levels. Because the amounts of various foods given in the Ultimate Family Food Guide reflect minimum amounts you and your family members can aim for each day to meet your nutrient and calorie needs, you can have more of your favorite foods (for example, pasta, red meat, or cheese) assuming you count those extra helpings as extra calories. If you buy a packaged item that bears a food label with calorie information on it, by all means use that. But because you may not have such information, see the following list for how to count extra calories when you help yourself to extra foods beyond the recommendations in your individual meal patterns:

- Fruit—If you have an extra ½ cup, count it as 60 extra calories.
- Vegetables—If you have an extra ½ cup of:
  Dark green, deep-yellow, and other vegetables, count it as 25 extra calories.
  Starchy vegetables, count it as 70 extra calories.
  Legumes (beans or peas), count it as 115 extra calories.

Extra Calories Based on Initial Calorie Level	
Calories	Extra Calories
900	100
1,000–1,400	150
1,600–1,800	200
2,000	250
2,200	300
2,400	350
2,600	400

- Grains—If you have an extra 1-ounce equivalent of grains, count it as 80 extra calories.
- Milk, yogurt, and cheese—If you have an extra 1-cup equivalent of milk, count it as 80 extra calories.
- Meat and beans—If you have an extra 1-ounce equivalent of meat and beans (excluding nuts and seeds and nut butters), count it as 55 extra calories; if you have an extra ½ ounce of nuts or seeds or 1 tablespoon of a nut butter, count it as 100 extra calories.
- Oils—If you have an extra teaspoon of oil, count it as 45 extra calories.

Foods and beverages that many of us consume but contain a lot of calories, fat, sugar, and few key nutrients include soft drinks, decadent coffee beverages, fruit drinks, and other caloric beverages (besides low-fat milk or 100% fruit juice). Candy, cookies, chips, butter, and cream cheese, just to name a few, also count as extra calories. Also, despite potential health benefits of small amounts of alcohol (red wine in particular), alcohol calories are counted as extra calories as well. See calorie counts for alcohol on page 168 and appendix G for foods that count as extra calories.

11

Preventing and Managing Diet-Related Conditions

Have you been diagnosed with or have a family history of any of the following?

- High blood cholesterol
- High triglycerides
- High blood pressure
- Diabetes—type 1, type 2, or gestational
- Hypoglycemia (low blood sugar)
- Metabolic syndrome
- Cancer
- Osteoporosis (fragile bones)

If you answered yes to any of these conditions, the good news is that there is much you and your family can do to manage and even prevent many of these diet-related diseases and conditions from occurring in the first place. For some families and some individuals, genes will undoubtedly overtake environment, but for most of us, how we eat, how we move, and how we live our lives will have a far greater effect than our genetic makeup on our health status and whether or not we develop diseases and conditions such as these. No matter what your current health status, following a meal pattern consistent with the Dietary Guidelines for Americans as described in chapter 10, as well as the meal plans highlighted in chapter 14, can help you move toward achieving a healthier body weight, and that alone can help you prevent a wide range of diet-related diseases and conditions. You can also use this chapter to better understand a variety of diet-related conditions or diseases you currently have or may be at risk for (list any conditions you and your family members have in the chart in appendix A). This chapter will show you and your family members how to fine-tune your dietary and lifestyle habits to manage or prevent such conditions. The information in this chapter is not meant to replace any advice or recommendations made by your doctor or any medications you may currently take. If you have any medical conditions or diseases, please consult your doctor and a registered dietitian before you make any changes in your dietary or lifestyle habits.

High Blood Cholesterol

Although it often gets a bad rap, cholesterol is vital to life and found in all cell membranes. It is necessary for the production of bile acids that help digestion as well as steroid hormones. Most of the cholesterol found in our blood is manufactured by our bodies at a rate of about 800 to 1,500 milligrams daily. The average American consumes between 300 and 450 milligrams of dietary cholesterol from food each day. When too much cholesterol and other substances build up in blood and accumulate in blood vessel walls, plaque forms in a process called atherosclerosis. This can ultimately reduce the flow of blood to the major arteries or cause blood clots; if blood vessels that lead to the heart or brain become blocked, the result can be a heart attack or stroke. Because atherosclerosis begins in childhood and progresses with age, it's a good idea to help kids develop healthful eating habits early on to reduce their risks when they're older. Controlling or preventing high blood cholesterol is one way to prevent the ill effects of atherosclerosis.

So what exactly is cholesterol? Cholesterol is not fat but rather a fat-like substance classified as a lipid. It travels through our blood via particles called lipoproteins, combinations of lipids and proteins. There are three major classes of lipoproteins: very low density lipoprotein (VLDL); low-density lipoprotein (LDL), which contains most of the cholesterol found in the blood; and high-density lipoprotein (HDL). LDL, often referred to as "bad cholesterol," seems to be the culprit in coronary heart disease. By contrast, HDL, known as "good cholesterol," is increasingly considered desirable because it is believed to carry the bad cholesterol out of the body.

To determine your lipoprotein levels—the levels of LDL cholesterol, total cholesterol, and HDL cholesterol in your blood—it is recommended that you have a blood test on an empty stomach (following a nine- to twelve-hour fast, without food, liquids, or pills). See "Counting Your Cholesterol" on this page or on page 120 to determine where you are in terms of your disease risk based on the numbers you obtain for your total, HDL, and LDL cholesterol levels.

Counting Your Cholesterol (in mg/dL): Adults

Total Cholesterol

    Less than 200 = desirable

    200–239 = borderline high risk

    240 and over = high risk

HDL Cholesterol

    Less than 40 for men and less than 50 for women = low HDL; a major risk factor for heart disease

    60 and above = high HDL; protective against heart disease

LDL Cholesterol

    Less than 100 = optimal

    100–129 = near or above optimal

    130–159 = borderline high

    160–189 = high

    190 and above = very high

Source: National Cholesterol Education Program, National Heart, Lung, and Blood Institute, National Institutes of Health, NIH Publication No. 01-3670, May 2001.

Your LDL goal depends on how many other risk factors you have. If you don't have coronary heart disease or diabetes and have one or no risk factors, your LDL goal is less than 160 mg/dL; if you don't have coronary heart disease or diabetes and have two or more risk factors, your LDL goal is less than 130 mg/dL; if you do have coronary heart disease or diabetes, your LDL goal is less than 100 mg/dL.

Some physicians and the American Heart Association recommend you use the ratio of *total* cholesterol to *HDL* cholesterol in place of just your total blood cholesterol as a quick estimate of your risks. You can determine the ratio by dividing your total cholesterol by your HDL cholesterol. For example, if you have a total cholesterol of 200 mg/dL and an HDL cholesterol level of 50 mg/dL, your ratio would be 4:1. The goal is to keep your ratio below 5:1; the optimum ratio is 3.5:1.

Following are guidelines from the National Cholesterol Education Program for cholesterol levels for children and adolescents between the ages of two and nineteen:

Counting Your Cholesterol (in mg/dL): Children and Teens

Total Cholesterol
Less than 170 = acceptable
170–199 = borderline
200 or greater = high

HDL Cholesterol
35 or greater = acceptable

LDL Cholesterol
Less than 110 = acceptable
110–129 = borderline
130 or greater = high

Source: National Cholesterol Education Program's Expert Panel on Blood Cholesterol in Children and Adolescents, 1991.

Because evidence indicates that elevated cholesterol levels early in life can lead to atherosclerosis (the buildup of harmful plaque), parents should help their children develop habits that promote healthful cholesterol levels to help prevent heart disease and other potential adverse health conditions that could otherwise occur later in life. Following an eating plan as described in chapter 10 and the family menu plans (see chapter 14) is a great first step toward maintaining normal blood cholesterol levels for all family members. Eating a diet rich in fruits and vegetables, curbing saturated fat to less than 10 percent of total calories, keeping trans fat intake as low as possible (less than 1 to 2 percent of total calories) can certainly help (see page 121 for daily limits for saturated fat and trans fat, and page 144 for food sources of each). Limiting dietary cholesterol to less than 300 milligrams per day can help (see page 121 for food sources). Not smoking, doing regular cardiovascu-

Daily Limits for Saturated Fat and Trans Fat*			
Initial Calorie Level	Less Than 10% of Total Calories from Saturated Fat Equals	Less Than 7% of Total Calories from Saturated Fat Equals	1 to 2% of Total Calories from Trans Fat Equals
1,000	Less than 11 g	Less than 8 g	1–2 g
1,200	Less than 13 g	Less than 9 g	1–2.5 g
1,400	Less than 16 g	Less than 11 g	1.5–3 g
1,600	Less than 18 g	Less than 12 g	2–3.5 g
1,800	Less than 20 g	Less than 14 g	2–4 g
2,000	Less than 22 g	Less than 16 g	2–4 g
2,200	Less than 24 g	Less than 17 g	2.5–5 g
2,400	Less than 27 g	Less than 19 g	2.5–5 g
2,600	Less than 29 g	Less than 20 g	3–6 g

*Amounts are approximate.

lar exercise, and achieving and maintaining a healthier body weight can, in many cases, help you prevent unhealthy cholesterol levels.

Unfortunately, some individuals develop high blood cholesterol levels largely because of a genetic predisposition and require more medications and a more restrictive dietary pattern to reduce their blood cholesterol levels significantly. These individuals, and those who already have high cholesterol levels mainly related to diet, may need to reduce their saturated fat intake to no more than 7 percent of total calories, and cholesterol intake to no more than 200 mg per day. See page 124 for tips to help you cut saturated fat and cholesterol from your diet. Increasing your intake of soluble

Top Sources of Dietary Cholesterol (from Most to Least)

Eggs

Beef

Poultry

Cheese

Milk

Fish/shellfish

Cakes/cookies/quick breads/doughnuts

Pork (fresh unprocessed)

Ice cream/sherbet/frozen yogurt

Sausage

Source: Dietary Guidelines 2005 Advisory Committee Report.

fiber from a variety of plant foods (10 to 25 grams per day; see food sources on page 122) can also have health benefits and further lower harmful LDL levels.

In addition to following a diet low in saturated fat, trans fat, and cholesterol and high in soluble fiber, those who have high total blood cholesterol and/or LDL cholesterol may further reduce their levels by adding 1 to 3 grams of plant sterols. These substances naturally occur in plant foods (such as oils, seeds, nuts, fruits, and vegetables), but the amounts in such foods are not always great enough to have a signifi-

Where's the Soluble Fiber?

Water-soluble fibers including pectin and gum are found inside plant cells. They slow down the rate at which food passes through the intestines. They can help lower blood cholesterol because they bind bile acids and can therefore increase the removal of cholesterol from the body. Following are some key food sources of soluble fiber (from most to least):

Food	Grams of Soluble Fiber
Psyllium seeds, ground (1 tablespoon)	5
Lima beans (½ cup cooked)	3.5
Brussels sprouts (½ cup cooked)	3
Kidney beans (½ cup cooked)	3
Orange, grapefruit (1 medium)	2
Pear (1 medium)	2
Black, navy, pinto beans (½ cup cooked)	2
Northern beans (½ cup cooked)	1.5
Prunes (¼ cup)	1.5
Apple, banana, nectarine, peach, plum (1 medium fruit)	1
Barley, oatmeal, or oat bran (½ cup)	1
Blackberries (½ cup)	1
Chickpeas, black-eyed peas (½ cup cooked)	1
Lentils (yellow, green, orange) (½ cup cooked)	1
Broccoli, carrots (½ cup cooked)	1

Source: Adapted from National Heart, Lung, and Blood Institute Soluble Fiber Tip Sheet.

cant blood-lowering effect. However, meeting your quota for fruits and vegetables (see chapter 10) and at the same time regularly consuming commercially prepared foods enriched with plant stanol or plant sterol esters (found in vegetable oil spreads like Benecol or Take Control, and/or low-fat yogurt or orange juice) in the recommended amounts can have significant total and LDL cholesterol–lowering effects. Dietary plant stanols and sterols are believed to inhibit cholesterol absorption in the small intestine by up to 50 percent, which in turn can lower LDL blood cholesterol by up to 14 percent. Even if you're already on medications such as statins to lower your blood cholesterol, plant stanols and sterols can further reduce your cholesterol levels because they work by a different mechanism.

High Triglycerides

Ninety-five percent of the lipids in food and in our bodies are triglycerides, which are fats. Many people develop high triglyceride levels as a consequence of an underlying disease such as uncontrolled diabetes, because they have kidney or thyroid problems, or because their diet is generally low in protein and high in refined carbohydrates. See the following guidelines to determine how your triglyceride levels stack up (after an overnight fast):

Triglyceride Level (in mg/dL): Adults
  Less than 150 mg/dL = normal
  150 to 199 mg/dL = borderline high
  200 to 499 mg/dL = high
  500 mg/dL or higher = very high

Triglyceride Level (in mg/dL): Children
  150 mg/dL or less = acceptable

You can lower your triglycerides or keep them within desirable levels by:

- Achieving or maintaining a healthy body weight
- Consuming foods that are low in saturated fat, trans fat, and cholesterol, and substituting foods high in saturated and trans fats with those high in monounsaturated and polyunsaturated fats; see "Fat Facts" on page 144 in chapter 12

- Substituting refined carbohydrates (especially sugary foods and beverages) with whole grains and unrefined carbohydrates
- Choosing fish in place of meats that are high in saturated fat and cholesterol; discuss fish oil supplements with your doctor (the American Heart Association recommends 2 to 4 grams of fish oil [EPA and DHA] a day for those with high blood triglycerides)
- Avoiding alcohol
- Avoiding cigarettes
- Getting regular exercise

Use the following tips to lower your intake of saturated fats, trans fat, and cholesterol when you buy, cook, and/or consume foods:

Healthier Heart Picks

Instead of:	Choose:
Solid fats (butter, shortening, or hard margarine)	Trans fat–free soft margarine, vegetable oils such as olive, canola, safflower, and sunflower
Fatty cuts of beef, chicken, and other meats	Lean cuts of beef, skinless white meat chicken and turkey breasts, and other lean cuts of meat
High-fat processed meats such as bacon, sausages, salami, and bologna	Low-fat, low-sodium meats (fresh or processed)
Eggs	Egg whites, egg substitutes
Full-fat or reduced-fat milk, yogurt, or cheese	1% or skim milk, low-fat yogurt, and low-fat cheese
Fried, breaded foods	Baked, steamed, boiled, broiled, or microwaved foods
Creamy and salty sauces	Seasoning with herbs and spices
Potato chips or corn chips, fried	Baked tortilla chips or air-popped popcorn, preferably unsalted

---

High Blood Pressure

Blood pressure is measured in two numbers. The top number is the systolic pressure, the pressure of blood in the vessels as the heart beats.

The lower number is the diastolic pressure, the pressure as the heart relaxes between heartbeats. High blood pressure, otherwise known as hypertension, is persistently elevated arterial blood pressure. It is the most common public health problem in developed countries. About 65 million Americans, or about 1 out of 3 adults age twenty and older, have high blood pressure. About 70 percent of those with high blood pressure know they have it (which means about 30 percent have it and don't know it; that's no surprise since in many cases, high blood pressure has no warning signs or symptoms). Having high blood pressure increases your risks for heart disease, kidney disease, and stroke. Anyone can develop high blood pressure. Once you develop high blood pressure, it usually doesn't go away; however, you can prevent and control high blood pressure by modifying your diet and lifestyle with or without medications. The table on this page will help you to get an idea of how your blood pressure stacks up if you're an adult.

Kids and Blood Pressure

Believe it or not, children are developing high blood pressure at earlier ages, which is no surprise given the rapid rise in the prevalence of obesity over recent decades. Your pediatrician can determine if your child has high blood pressure by taking a measurement on at least three separate occasions and comparing it with blood pressure standards for children based on gender, age, and height that classify blood pressure according to body size. Children and adolescents with blood pressure levels at or above 120/80 mmHg but below the ninety-fifth percentile should be considered prehypertensive. Because high blood pressure in

Blood Pressure: What Do Your Numbers Mean?		
Blood Pressure Classification	Systolic Blood Pressure (the top number, in mmHg)	Diastolic Blood Pressure (the bottom number, in mmHg)
Normal	Less than 120	and less than 80
Pre-hypertension	120–139	or 80–89
Stage 1 hypertension	140–159	or 90–99
Stage 2 hypertension	160 and above	100 and above

Source: National Cholesterol Education Program.

children can produce long-term health risks similar to those faced by adults who develop the condition, it's important for parents and their pediatricians to help children develop healthful eating and physical activity habits to support adequate but not excessive growth in terms of body weight.

Preventing or Managing High Blood Pressure

Although the causes of high blood pressure are not fully understood, having family members with high blood pressure can increase your risk for developing the condition as well. In addition, many environmental contributors work alone or in concert to promote the development of high blood pressure. They include consuming few fruits and vegetables, too much sodium and salt, too much alcohol, not enough low-fat dairy foods, not getting enough physical activity, smoking, older age, having uneven hormone levels or abnormalities in the nervous and circulatory systems and kidneys, having conditions that make you retain too much salt and water in your body for whatever reason, taking birth control pills, or being an African American. No matter what the contributors, there are several steps you can take in terms of your diet and lifestyle to lower your blood pressure. If you have high blood pressure, discuss diet and medications with your doctor before making any changes in your current habits. The recommendations in chapter 10 and exercise tips in chapter 3 can help you prevent or manage high blood pressure. Losing weight, engaging in regular physical activity, eating a diet rich in fruits, vegetables, low-fat dairy foods, and nuts and seeds, restricting dietary sodium (see the list of tips from the 2005 Dietary Guidelines Advisory Committee Report on this page; you may need to go as low as 1,500 milligrams per day—discuss this with your physician), limiting alcoholic beverages, and avoiding smoking are all helpful in lowering your blood pressure if it's high or preventing high blood pressure from occurring in the first place.

Top Tips to Lower Your Sodium Intake

At the store:

- Choose fresh or plain frozen vegetables (they are naturally low in salt), or canned vegetables without added salt.
- Choose fresh or frozen fish, shellfish, poultry, and meat. They are lower in salt than most canned and processed forms.

- Read Nutrition Facts panels to compare the amount of sodium in processed foods such as frozen dinners, packaged mixes, cereals, cheese, breads, soups, salad dressings, and sauces. The amount in different types and brands often varies widely.
- Look for labels that say low sodium. They contain 140 milligrams (about 5 percent of the Daily Value) or less of sodium per serving.
- Ask your grocer or supermarket to offer more low-sodium foods.

Cooking and eating at home:

- If you add salt to foods when cooking or at the table, add small amounts. Learn to use spices and herbs, rather than salt, to enhance the flavor of food.
- Go easy on condiments such as soy sauce, ketchup, mustard, pickles, and olives; they can add a lot of salt to your food.
- Leave the salt shaker in a cupboard.

Eating out:

- Choose plain foods like grilled or roasted entrées, baked potatoes, and salad with oil and vinegar. Batter-fried foods tend to be high in salt, as are combination dishes like stews or pasta with sauce.
- Ask to have no salt added when the food is prepared.

Any time:

- Choose fruits and vegetables often.
- Drink water freely. It is usually very low in sodium. Check the label on bottled water for sodium content.

The DASH Diet

The DASH (Dietary Approaches to Stop Hypertension) Diet, supported and sponsored by the National Institutes of Health, is now part of the official high blood pressure guidelines in the United States and abroad. It is also incorporated into the *Dietary Guidelines for Americans 2005*. In a carefully controlled program, the multicenter study involving 800 participants and 80 physicians proved the effectiveness of diet in lowering blood pressure. Some participants were placed on a typical American diet and others ate the DASH diet full of fruits, vegetables, and low-salt food. The DASH diet lowered blood pressure in DASH study participants by an average of 5.5 mmHg (systolic) and 3 mmHg (diastolic). Reductions in blood pressure occurred within a week of starting the diet, stabilized within two weeks, and stayed the same for the remaining six weeks of the study. In those participants with high blood pressure, the DASH diet dramatically lowered blood pressure an average of 11.4 mmHg (systolic) and 5.5 mmHg (diastolic).

The majority of people who have high blood pressure are predisposed to the disease because it runs in the family, according to the landmark U.S. study. However, some people who are not predisposed to hypertension may develop the disease simply because of their dietary and lifestyle habits. But even if you have a family history of hypertension, a healthy diet and lifestyle may protect you against developing it.

Diabetes

Diabetes is the name used to describe a group of medical disorders characterized by high blood sugar levels. Normally when you eat, your food is digested and much of it is converted to glucose, simple sugars that are your body's key source of energy. Your blood carries glucose to your cells where it is absorbed with the help of the hormone insulin. If you have diabetes, however, your body does not make enough insulin or cannot properly use the insulin it does make. Without insulin, glucose accumulates in your blood rather than moving into your cells, and you develop high blood sugar levels.

More than 18 million Americans are estimated to have diabetes today. That's an increase of over 45 percent since just a decade ago according to the American Medical Association. African Americans, Mexican Americans, and Native Americans have experienced a particularly sharp rise in the prevalence of type 2 diabetes in the past decade. National statistics show that deaths from heart disease, stroke, and cancer are down, but deaths from diabetes are on the rise as are severe complications related to diabetes. Diabetes is the number-one cause of adult blindness in the United States, the leading cause of end-stage kidney disease, and the primary cause of nontraumatic amputation. So far there is no cure, but it is a condition that can be dramatically controlled through diet, exercise, and medication.

The Types of Diabetes

Following are three distinct forms of diabetes that a person can develop.

Type 1 Diabetes

This form of diabetes was previously called insulin-dependent diabetes mellitus (IDDM) or juvenile-onset diabetes. Type 1 diabetes develops when the body's immune system destroys pancreatic beta cells, the only cells in the body that make insulin. This form of diabetes usually strikes children and young adults, although disease onset can occur at any age. Type 1 diabetes may account for 5 to 10 percent of all diagnosed cases of diabetes. Risk factors for type 1 diabetes may include autoimmune, genetic, and environmental factors.

Type 2 Diabetes

This form of diabetes was previously called non-insulin-dependent diabetes mellitus (NIDDM) or adult-onset diabetes. Type 2 diabetes may account for about 90 to 95 percent of all diagnosed cases of diabetes. It usually begins as insulin resistance, a disorder in which the cells do not use insulin properly. As the need for insulin rises, the pancreas gradually loses its ability to produce insulin. Type 2 diabetes is associated with older age, obesity, family history of diabetes, history of gestational diabetes, impaired glucose metabolism, physical inactivity, and race/ethnicity. African Americans, Hispanic/Latino Americans, Native Americans, and some Asian Americans and Native Hawaiians or other Pacific Islanders are at particularly high risk for type 2 diabetes. Although type 2 diabetes used to be known as an adult disease, it is increasingly being diagnosed in children and adolescents, which is no surprise given the surge in overweight among this population in recent years.

Gestational Diabetes

This condition is a form of glucose intolerance diagnosed in some women during pregnancy. Gestational diabetes occurs more frequently among African Americans, Hispanic/Latino Americans, and Native Americans. It is also more common among obese women and women with a family history of diabetes. During pregnancy, gestational diabetes requires treatment to normalize maternal blood glucose levels to avoid complications in the infant. After pregnancy, 5 to 10 percent of women with gestational diabetes are found to have type 2 diabetes.

Women who have had gestational diabetes have a 20 to 50 percent chance of developing diabetes in the next five to ten years.

Other specific types of diabetes result from specific genetic conditions (such as maturity-onset diabetes of youth), surgery, drugs, malnutrition, infections, and other illnesses. Such types of diabetes may account for 1 to 5 percent of all diagnosed cases of diabetes.

Testing for Diabetes

To see whether or not you have prediabetes or diabetes, your healthcare provider may conduct a fasting plasma glucose (FPG) test or an oral glucose tolerance test (OGTT). Although either test can be used, the American Diabetes Association recommends the FPG because it's faster and less expensive to perform.

- FPG test—a value of 100 and 125 mg/dL signals prediabetes; a value of 126 mg/dL or higher signals diabetes.
- OGTT—In this test, a person's blood glucose level is measured after a fast and two hours after drinking a glucose-rich beverage. If the two-hour blood glucose level is between 140 and 199 mg/dL, the person tested has prediabetes. If the two-hour blood glucose level is at 200 mg/dL, the person tested has diabetes.

Prediabetes is a condition in which blood glucose levels are higher than normal but not high enough for a diagnosis of diabetes. About 41 million Americans are estimated to have prediabetes, according to the National Institute of Diabetes and Kidney and Digestive Diseases (NIDKD). People with prediabetes have an increased risk of developing type 2 diabetes, heart disease, and stroke. Prediabetes is sometimes called impaired fasting glucose (IFG) or impaired glucose tolerance (IGT), depending on the test used to diagnose it. IFG is a condition in which the fasting blood glucose level is elevated (100 to 125 mg/dL) after an overnight fast but is not high enough to be classified as diabetes. IGT is a condition in which the blood glucose level is elevated (140 to 199 mg/dL) after a two-hour oral glucose tolerance test but is not high enough to be classified as diabetes. Some people have both IFG and IGT.

Preventing Diabetes through Diet and Exercise

According to the NIDKD, lifestyle changes can prevent or delay the onset of type 2 diabetes among high-risk adults. These studies included people who had IGT and other high-risk characteristics for developing diabetes. Lifestyle interventions included diet and moderate-intensity physical activity (such as walking for 2½ hours each week). In the Diabetes Prevention Program, a large prevention study of people at high risk for diabetes, the development of diabetes was reduced 58 percent over three years.

As you have read, progression to diabetes if you have prediabetes is not inevitable. Studies suggest that if you have prediabetes, weight loss and increased physical activity can prevent or delay diabetes and may return your blood glucose levels to normal. Following an eating plan consistent with the guide in chapter 10 based on the Dietary Guidelines for Americans 2005 is a great place to start whether you have diabetes or wish to prevent it. Studies have shown that having three 1-ounce equivalents of whole grains and about 1 ounce of nuts a day, choosing fish high in omega-3 fats or having fish oil (discuss with your physician), and exercising can promote optimal health and possibly play a role in reducing your risk for type 2 diabetes.

You do not have to avoid sugar entirely. A little bit is okay, but of course you want to limit refined grains, emphasize healthful whole grains, fruits, and vegetables, and maintain an optimal and balanced overall dietary pattern. People with diabetes may want to use their extra calories from foods rich in monounsaturated and polyunsaturated fats instead of from refined or sugary foods to promote more stable blood sugar levels throughout the day. Losing excess weight and, in some cases, oral medications can also help people manage and in some cases even reverse their diabetes.

Hypoglycemia (Low Blood Sugar)

Hypoglycemia is a condition in which your blood glucose (blood sugar) drops too low to provide enough energy for your body's activities. Glucose, a form of sugar, is an important fuel for your brain and body. Carbohydrate-rich foods such as potatoes, rice, pasta, breads, cereals, fruits, and vegetables provide dietary sources of glucose. After a meal, glucose molecules are absorbed into your bloodstream and carried to the cells, where they are used for energy. Insulin, a hormone produced by your pancreas, helps glucose enter cells. If you take in more glucose than your body needs at the time, your body stores the extra glucose in your liver and muscles in a form called glycogen. Your body can use the stored glucose whenever it is needed for energy between meals. Extra glucose can also be converted to fat and stored in fat cells.

When your blood glucose begins to fall, glucagon, another hormone produced by your pancreas, signals your liver to break down glycogen and release glucose, causing your blood glucose levels to rise toward a normal level. If you have diabetes, this glucagon response to hypoglycemia may be impaired, making it harder for your glucose levels to return to the normal range. Symptoms of low blood sugar include:

- Hunger
- Nervousness and shakiness
- Perspiration
- Dizziness or light-headedness
- Sleepiness
- Confusion
- Difficulty speaking
- Feeling anxious or weak
- Crying out or having nightmares while sleeping
- Finding pajamas or sheets damp from perspiration
- Feeling tired, irritable, or confused when waking up

The following will help you determine how your blood sugar level stacks up. Normal and target blood glucose ranges are in mg/dL:

- Normal blood glucose levels in people who do not have diabetes:
    Upon waking (fasting): 70–110
    After meals: 70–140
- Target blood glucose levels in people who have diabetes:
    Before meals: 90–130
    1 to 2 hours after the start of a meal: less than 180
- Hypoglycemia (low blood glucose):
    70 or below

Serious low blood sugar is usually a side effect of diabetes treatment, but according to the NIDKD at the National Institutes of Health some medications, or hormone or enzyme deficiencies may cause low blood sugar. A drop in blood sugar may also occur occasionally in healthy people who may skip meals, load up on carbohydrate-rich foods, or overdo physical activity.

If you have any form of diabetes or prediabetes, talk to your physician or a health-care professional about whether you should have a snack or adjust your medication before sports or exercise. If you know you will be more active than usual or will be doing something that is not part of your normal routine—shoveling snow, for example—consider having a snack first. Drinking alcoholic beverages, especially on an empty stomach, can cause hypoglycemia, even a day or two later. If you drink an alcoholic beverage, always have a snack or meal at the same time to minimize the alcohol's effects.

Keep your blood sugar as close to the normal range as possible to reduce potential long-term complications from high or low blood sugar. If you have any problem stabilizing your blood sugar, be sure to consult with your physician and meet with a registered dietitian who can help you create your own individualized healthy eating plan. The Ultimate Family Food Guide (see chapter 10) and meal plans (see chapter 14) can help you get started on a healthier eating course. In addition, people with hypoglycemia want to make sure to have regular, frequent meals, include protein-rich foods from the meat and beans and/or the milk/yogurt/cheese food categories and minimize refined foods including sugary foods and beverages.

Metabolic Syndrome

This syndrome refers to a cluster of the most dangerous risk factors for a heart attack: diabetes and prediabetes, abdominal obesity, high blood cholesterol, and high blood pressure. An estimated 1 in 4 adults in the world has metabolic syndrome, which makes them twice as likely to die from and three times as likely to have a heart attack or stroke compared with those without the syndrome. They also have five times the risk of developing type 2 diabetes.

According to the National Heart, Lung, and Blood Institute's 2001 report *National Cholesterol Education Program: Third Report of the Expert Panel on Detection, Evaluation, and Treatment of High Blood Cholesterol in Adults*, metabolic syndrome is defined by the presence of any three of the following conditions:

- Excess weight around the waist (waist measurement of more than 40 inches for men and more than 35 inches for women)
- High levels of triglycerides (150 mg/dL or higher)

- Low levels of HDL, or good cholesterol (below 40 mg/dL for men and below 50 mg/dL for women)
- Blood pressure readings of 130/85 mmHg or higher
- Fasting blood glucose levels (110 mg/dL or higher)

You may be able to tell whether you may have metabolic syndrome merely by measuring your waistline. People with abdominal obesity are at serious risk of insulin resistance, an early stage in the development of diabetes and heart disease, according to a study published by the *British Medical Journal*. Because there is no easy test to predict the insulin resistance of an individual, Swedish researchers set out to assess the ability of different body measurements and biological markers to predict insulin sensitivity. Their study involved 2,746 healthy male and female volunteers between the ages of eighteen and seventy-two years with BMIs from 18 and 60 kg/m^2 and waist circumferences from 65 to 150 centimeters. Height, weight, waist, and hip circumference were measured, and a blood sample was taken to determine insulin sensitivity. The researchers found that waist circumference was a very strong independent predictor of insulin sensitivity as in type 2 diabetes, prediabetes, and metabolic syndrome. A waist circumference of less than 100 centimeters excluded insulin resistance in both sexes. The authors believe that waist circumference is better than BMI, waist-to-hip ratio, and other measures of total body fat as a predictor of insulin resistance. Other research has found that waist circumference is associated with insulin resistance in children as well and provides a simple way to identify children with risk factors for cardiovascular disease and type 2 diabetes.

The recommended treatment for metabolic syndrome includes weight loss and increased physical activity and treating conditions that may be present (including high LDL cholesterol levels—see page 118, high triglycerides—see page 123, and high blood pressure—see page 124).

The Ultimate Family Food Guide in chapter 10, the exercise recommendations in chapter 3, and all the tips in this book can help you and your family members achieve and maintain a healthier body weight and help you prevent or at least reduce your chances for developing metabolic syndrome and related conditions.

Cancer

Cancer is the general term used for more than one hundred different diseases. Dietary factors are estimated to account for approximately 30 percent of cancers that occur in Western countries, making diet second only to tobacco as a preventable cause of cancer. This proportion is thought to be about 20 percent in developing countries and projected to grow. As developing countries become urbanized, patterns of cancer, particularly those most strongly associated with diet and physical activity, tend to shift toward the patterns of more economically developed countries. Cancer rates also change as populations move between countries and adopt different dietary patterns.

The Connection among Cancer, Diet, and Physical Activity

Although cancer certainly has strong genetic components in many families, major environmental contributors play a role in cancer. The table on page 136 from the World Health Organization summarizes the strength of evidence on lifestyle factors and the risk of developing cancer.

Strategies to Reduce Cancer Risk

Following a meal pattern consistent with the Ultimate Family Food Guide, based on the Dietary Guidelines for Americans 2005 (see chapter 10), and the menus in chapter 14 is a great starting point for preventing cancer and other adverse health conditions associated with diet. Here are some other general tips adapted from those of the World Health Organization to help you and your family reduce your risk for developing cancer during your lifetime:

- Maintain a healthy body weight for life; prevent excess weight gain during early childhood through adolescence and prevent weight gain through your adult years.
- Maintain a regular, consistent physical activity pattern throughout life. Staying active during your leisure time and doing formal physical activity on all or most days can help you burn calories to help you achieve or maintain a healthier body weight, build or preserve muscle mass, and keep your heart strong.

Evidence for the Role of Diet and Lifestyle in Cancer Prevention and Promotion		
Evidence	**Decreased Risk**	**Increased Risk**
Convincing	Physical activity (colon, breast)	Overweight and obesity (esophagus, colorectum, breast in postmenopausal women, endometrium, kidney); alcohol (oral cavity, pharynx, larynx, esophagus, liver, breast); aflatoxin (liver); Chinese-style salted fish (nasopharynx)
Probable	Fruits and vegetables (oral cavity, esophagus, stomach, colorectum)[a] Physical activity (breast)	Preserved meat (colorectum); salt-preserved foods, and salt (stomach); very hot (temperature) drinks and food (oral cavity, pharynx, esophagus)
Possible/ insufficient	Fiber, soy, fish, omega-3 fatty acids, carotenoids, vitamin B_2, B_6, folate, B_{12}, C, D, E, calcium, zinc, selenium, nonnutrient plant constituents (for example, allium compounds, lignins, flavonoids, isoflavones)	Animal fats, heterocyclic amines, polycyclic aromatic hydrocarbons, and nitrosamines.[b]

Source: The World Health Organization, Global Strategy on Diet, Physical Activity and Health: Cancer, 2003.

[a] For colorectal cancer, a protective effect of fruit and vegetable intake is suggested by many case-control studies, but has not been supported by results of several large prospective studies, suggesting that if a benefit does exist it is likely to be modest.

[b] The food-derived heterocyclic amines (HCAs) comprise a family of mutagenic/carcinogenic compounds found in a variety of meats that are cooked by ordinary household methods.

- Avoid alcohol; if you do consume it, limit it to no more than one drink per day for women and two drinks per day for men (one drink is defined as 12 ounces of beer, 5 ounces of table wine, or 1½ ounces of distilled spirits).

- Limit your consumption of salt-preserved foods (such as Chinese-style fermented salted fish) and table salt as much as possible.
- Minimize exposure to aflatoxins in food (aflatoxins are poisonous substances that can grow in improperly stored nuts, grains, dried fruits, spices, and certain other foods).
- Consume a diet rich in fruits, vegetables, whole grains, beans, peas, and lentils.
- Those who are not vegetarian are advised to moderate consumption of preserved meat (for example, sausages, salami, bacon, and ham).
- Do not consume foods or drinks when they are at a very hot (scalding) temperature.

Osteoporosis

Osteoporosis is a skeletal disease in which the bones lose mass and density, the pores in bones enlarge, and the bones generally become fragile. Osteoporosis is not usually diagnosed until a fracture occurs, most commonly in the spine, hip, or wrist. It is another condition that has a strong dietary component, especially as it relates to women and young girls.

Osteoporosis affects more than 25 million Americans, mostly women past menopause. Approximately 1.2 million bone fractures each year in the United States are related to osteoporosis. The National Osteoporosis Foundation says that 1 in 2 women and 1 in 8 men over the age of fifty will have an osteoporosis-related fracture in their lifetime. Thirty-three percent of women over the age of sixty-five will experience a fracture of the spine, and as many as 20 percent of hip fracture patients will die within six months from conditions caused by lack of activity such as blood clots and pneumonia. Throughout life, bones go through a constant state of loss and growth. As people age, however, they lose bone at a more rapid rate, and osteoporosis may develop. Osteoporosis causes the bones to become thin and fragile, increasing the chance of breaking with even minor injury.

Healthful dietary and exercise habits early in life may strengthen bones and thus delay the development of osteoporosis in later life. Studies show that exercising during teenage years can increase bone mass and greatly reduce the risk of osteoporosis in adulthood. The best type of exercise to build bones is weight-bearing exercise, like walking or stair climbing, and weight or resistance training (see chapter 3 for more about exercise). Even if you develop osteoporosis, consuming adequate calcium and vitamin D from food sources and, in some cases, dietary supplements (be sure to discuss this with your physician, especially if you don't consume adequate amounts of calcium and vitamin D–rich foods and beverages, including nondairy sources of calcium) can retard the process and reduce the risk of bone fractures. See appendix D for calcium and vitamin D needs and key food sources. See the following tips for ways to increase your daily calcium intake:

- Aim for two to three 1-cup equivalents of milk/cheese/yogurt each day to maximize your daily calcium intake.
- Include several nondairy sources of calcium each day including dark green vegetables, beans and seeds, fish with bones, and other foods (see appendix D for a list of nondairy food sources of calcium).
- Use low-fat or nonfat dairy products to cut calories and to keep the amount of fat in the diet at recommended levels. Add ⅓ cup to ½ cup nonfat dry milk powder to recipes for pancakes, breads, mashed potatoes, scrambled eggs, puddings, cookies, cakes, and other foods. The milk powder can be blended into the other dry ingredients (flour, sugar, and so on) or added along with the water or liquid milk.
- Substitute low-fat yogurt for sour cream or mayonnaise in recipes, dips, dressings, and toppings.
- Choose spinach, romaine, and other dark-colored salad greens instead of iceberg lettuce when you make a salad.
- Use low-fat milk or low-fat buttermilk instead of water to reconstitute canned soups, dry cereal such as Cream of Wheat, instant mashed potatoes, and salad dressing mixes.
- Consume low-fat pudding, frozen yogurt, ice cream, and custard to get some added calcium at snack or dessert time.
- Add nonfat dry milk powder to skim or 1% milk; adding an extra ⅓ cup of dry milk powder per 1 cup liquid milk will double the calcium content and make the milk richer without altering the taste.
- Add milk or evaporated milk to coffee instead of cream. Or, for convenience, use nonfat dry milk powder rather than nondairy creamer.

- Mix lemon juice, a few drops of olive oil, crushed garlic, and grated Parmesan cheese for a low-calorie, high-calcium salad dressing.
- Top casseroles, omelets, toast, baked potatoes, and steamed vegetables with shredded cheddar, Swiss, or mozzarella cheese for a calcium boost.
- Add tofu with added calcium to salads and stir-fries.
- If you limit your intake of dairy foods, look for calcium-fortified versions of products you already buy, such as orange juice, low-fat hot chocolate mix, pancake mix, and other foods.

Vitamin D is essential in order to absorb calcium from foods. Besides sunlight, other sources are vitamin D–fortified margarines and dairy products, fortified breakfast cereals, and oily fish. Because it's challenging to get adequate vitamin D from foods alone, some researchers recommend vitamin D supplements, especially for older people, those with dark skin, and those who don't get adequate sunlight from the outdoors. If you think you may be a candidate for vitamin D supplements, be sure to discuss this with your physician.

In addition to boosting your calcium and vitamin D intake and getting plenty of regular exercise, the 2004 *Surgeon General's Report on Bone Health and Osteoporosis* recommends other strategies to protect bones, including maintaining a healthy body weight, not smoking, and limiting or abstaining from alcohol. These strategies are also quite effective in helping you ward off obesity and overweight and many chronic diseases and conditions including those discussed in this chapter.

In addition to getting adequate calcium and vitamin D, recent research from the Centre for Nutrition and Food Safety in the United Kingdom has found a positive link between vegetable and fruit consumption and bone health. Women who had consumed the most fruit during childhood were found to have higher bone mineral density than those who reported eating less fruit. Because of its emphasis on fruits and vegetables, whole grains, low-fat dairy foods, and lean protein sources, following a dietary pattern consistent with the Dietary Guidelines for Americans 2005 as detailed in chapter 10 and the family meal plans in chapter 14 can help you stave off osteoporosis. This dietary pattern will not only benefit your bones but reduce your overall disease risks and improve your nutrient intake to keep you and your family healthy and strong.

I hope this chapter has convinced you that even if you or your family members have a disease or condition, there is much you can do in terms of your dietary and lifestyle behaviors to affect your health positively. Whether it's to prevent or treat/manage a diet-related condition, all the information throughout this book can help educate and inspire you and your family to adopt more healthful dietary and lifestyle behaviors.

12

Surviving the Grocery Aisles

Going to the grocery store, especially with a child (or children) in tow, can be a daunting task. If you're like most families, you are time starved as it is, and reading food labels and comparing products may not be realistic for you to do most of the time. This chapter will give you some shortcuts and quick tips to help you navigate unscathed through grocery store aisles and fill your cart with nourishing foods your entire family will enjoy and that will please multiple palates.

Before you venture out to restock your kitchen with food, take some time to see where you're starting from and where you're headed.

Step 1: Raid the refrigerator. Make a list of anything and everything that's edible in your refrigerator. Also, go through your freezer, pantry, and even the cookie jar or other food containers on your counter. Taking stock of what's in your kitchen will help you:

- Determine what has already expired or spoiled (see the resources at the end of the book for food safety information).
- See what you and your family are really eating. Are most of the foods in your pantry salty, fatty snacks like chips or sweet treats like candy and cookies, and is your refrigerator packed with sugary sodas and fruit drinks? Are there few fruits and vegetables from which to choose? Is your freezer filled with ice cream and high-fat frozen French fries and waffles?

- Decide what types of foods and beverages you and your family need more of, and which ones you need less of to meet your nutrient needs and promote healthy weights (see "Survival in the Aisles Guide" beginning on page 146 for tips to help you make more healthful selections from the key food categories as described in chapter 10).

Step 2: Make a list. The Ultimate Family Food Shopping List on page 155 contains all the items listed in the two weeks of menus (see chapter 14) as well as the recipes included in those menus (see chapter 15). You can photocopy this list to use each week, or use it as a template to make your own personalized list. Check off any items you already have (for example, olive oil or other staples), and highlight or circle those items to buy.

Step 3: Eat before you shop. It's true that when you're hungry, you're much more likely to cave into cravings brought on by the sight or smell of appealing food. To reduce the likelihood that you'll be lured by the smell of chocolate cake or buttery brioche in the bakery section, or the candy bars stacked up near the checkout lines, eat at least a small snack to tide you over before you go. If your kids are in tow as well, you can keep small plastic bags with some dry whole-grain cereal, whole-grain crackers, or a small box of raisins to offer if and when hunger strikes.

The Food Label Decoded

When you shop for food and other items, the Nutrition Facts panel, or food label, can be quite useful. Knowing how to read a food label is key for families who want to make more informed and healthful selections from among the seemingly limitless options available at today's supermarkets. Teaching kids how to read food labels at an early age gives them the know-how to make healthier choices when they buy food away from home.

Most foods and beverages, including breads, cereals, canned and frozen foods, snacks, desserts, and drinks, are required by law to bear food labels. But some foods—raw fruits and vegetables, and fish—are not required to have food labels, although they may voluntarily have them. Next is a brief description of the key information provided on food labels, followed by an aisle-by-aisle guide (see page 146) to help you make healthier selections from all the food categories emphasized in chapter 10.

Servings

Serving size is listed at the top of the label. This tells you how much of the item equals one serving, or one portion. All the information about calories and nutrients listed on the label is for one serving. If you have two servings of any item, you'll need to double the calories and other nutrients listed on the label to know exactly how much you're getting. *Servings per container* are also listed to let you know how many servings are in the entire package. If there are ten servings in a box of crackers and each serving is five crackers, then the box will contain about fifty crackers.

Nutrition Facts

Serving Size 1 cup (228g)
Servings Per Container 2

Amount Per Serving

Calories 260   Calories from Fat 120

	% Daily Value*
Total Fat 13g	**20%**
Saturated Fat 5g	**25%**
Trans Fat 0g	
Cholesterol 30mg	**10%**
Sodium 660mg	**28%**
Total Carbohydrate 31g	**10%**
Dietary Fiber 0g	**0%**
Sugars 5g	
Protein 5g	

Vitamin A 4%	•	Vitamin C 2%
Calcium 15%	•	Iron 4%

* Percent Daily Values are based on a 2,000 calorie diet. Your Daily Values may be higher or lower depending on your calorie needs:

		Calories:	2,000	2,500
Total Fat	Less than		65g	80g
Sat Fat	Less than		20g	25g
Cholesterol	Less than		300mg	300mg
Sodium	Less than		2,400mg	2,400mg
Total Carbohydrate			300g	375g
Dietary Fiber			25g	30g

Calories per gram:
Fat 9   •   Carbohydrate 4   •   Protein 4

Calories and Calories from Fat

Calories per serving tells you how much energy is in the food. To manage your weight, look at calories and think about how they fit into your total calorie intake for the day. For example, if you require about 1,600 calories a day and would like to snack on some whole-grain crackers, ten crackers equals one serving and have 160 calories; those crackers alone make up 10 percent of your total calories for the day.

Calories from fat are also listed. If an item has 200 calories, and 150 of the calories come from fat, that's considered a high-fat food.

Total Fat, Saturated Fat, and Trans Fats

Total fat is listed in grams; it includes saturated fat, trans fat, mono-unsaturated fats, and polyunsaturated fats that can be found in foods. At minimum, products are required by law to list saturated fat and trans fat under total fat on food labels. Monounsaturated fat and polyunsaturated fat may or may not be listed. Although fat has many key functions—it helps our bodies absorb and transport fat-sol-uble vitamins (vitamins A, D, E, and K) around the body and insu-lates our bodies to protect organs and tissues and maintain body temperature—we need to pay attention to how much fat we eat and the type of fat we choose. Most of us should aim for 20 to 35 percent of total calories from fat each day. That's about 38 to 56 grams for someone who consumes 1,600 calories a day. Most of the fat we con-sume should come from monounsaturated and polyunsaturated sources, and ideally less than 12 percent of total calories should come from saturated and trans fats combined (see the table on page 121). People with heart disease or high blood cholesterol levels should aim for no more than 7 percent of total calories from saturated fats and trans fats combined. Fat is very energy dense (it has 9 calories per

Fat Facts		
Type of Fat	**Key Food Sources**	**Health Effects**
Saturated fat	Butter, whole milk, and products made with whole milk (including ice cream and cheese), red meats, chocolate, coconut, and products made with coconut	Raises total cholesterol as well as bad LDL cholesterol levels.
Trans fat	Many margarines, partially hydrogenated vegetable oils; fried snack chips; commercial baked goods such as cakes, cookies, doughnuts, and cupcakes; breaded frozen foods and frozen breakfast foods such as waffles and pancakes; small amounts found naturally in some animal foods, including meats and high fat dairy foods	Raises total cholesterol and bad LDL cholesterol; it also lowers good HDL cholesterol levels.
Monounsaturated fat	Olive oil, canola oil, peanut oil, nuts (including almonds, cashews, and peanuts), olives, and avocados	When used to replace saturated fats, can lower total cholesterol and bad LDL cholesterol.
Polyunsaturated fat	Corn oil, soybean oil, safflower oil, sunflower oil, and fish oil	When used to replace saturated fats, can lower total cholesterol and bad LDL cholesterol.

gram versus 4 calories per gram for both protein and carbohydrate). Because fat calories can add up quickly, it's important to keep an eye on how much fat you consume, even if the fat sources you choose are mostly healthful.

Cholesterol

Cholesterol is listed in milligrams. It is a type of fat found in all animal foods and foods made with animal foods such as milk or butter. Our bodies make most of the cholesterol in our blood, but we absorb about 20 to 25 percent of the cholesterol from the food we consume. Even though saturated fat and trans fat have a great impact on blood cholesterol levels, it's important to watch cholesterol intake because too much cholesterol in your blood can increase your risk for heart disease. The Dietary Guidelines for Americans 2005 recommend that we keep our cholesterol intake to no more than 300 milligrams per day; those who have heart disease or high blood cholesterol are encouraged to aim for no more than 200 milligrams per day.

Sodium

Sodium is listed in milligrams. The Dietary Guidelines for Americans 2005 recommend no more than 2,300 milligrams per day (up to 1,500 milligrams for those who have high blood pressure or are salt sensitive).

Total Carbohydrate

Total carbohydrate is listed in grams. Carbohydrate provides the body, including the brain and the central nervous system, with its chief source of fuel. Dietary fiber and sugars, each in grams, are also listed under total carbohydrate. Dietary fiber is important to maintain proper bowel function and healthy cholesterol levels. Fiber is also quite filling, and most high-fiber foods contain other healthful nutrients and are low in calories and/or fat. Fiber needs vary depending on your age, but most Americans need to double up on their current fiber intake to achieve recommended levels (see appendix D for adults; children can likely meet their fiber needs by consuming whole grains, fruits, and vegetables as recommended in chapter 10). Sugars provide calories but not much else (see "Hidden Sugars," page 153).

Protein

Protein is listed in grams. Protein is needed to build and repair body tissues including muscle and bone. Most people consume enough or too much protein, but they don't always choose the leanest, most nutrient-dense forms (see chapter 10 for tips to make healthier protein picks).

Vitamin A, Vitamin C, Calcium, and Iron

The amounts of these key vitamins and minerals are listed in percentages. Because many Americans don't get enough of these key nutrients (see appendix D for your individual needs), food labels show how much of these nutrients a product contributes compared with daily values for those nutrients (based on an adult who follows a 2,000-calorie diet). For example, if a product lists 15 percent for calcium, that means it provides 15 percent of a person's daily calcium needs.

Survival in the Aisles Guide

The following is a guide to help you and your family make more healthful choices when you shop for foods and beverages that fit into your healthy eating plan.

Fruits

When you buy fruit, make sure it's in its lowest sugar form. Following are some additional tips to help you make more healthful fruit selections:

- Fresh fruit. Choose whatever fruits you love! Here are some superstars in terms of fiber, vitamins, minerals, and antioxidants (note that some of these may also be found frozen or canned):

  Fiber—figs, oranges, raspberries, pears, blackberries, mangoes, kiwis, peaches, and bananas

  Vitamin A—mangoes, cantaloupes, and apricots

  Vitamin C—guavas, papayas, oranges, and orange juice

  Folate—oranges and orange juice

  Potassium—bananas, plantains, oranges, and many dried fruits

  Antioxidants—blueberries, blackberries, prunes, raspberries, strawberries, cranberries, apples, sweet cherries, and plums

- Frozen fruit. Look for unsweetened frozen fruit.

- Canned fruit. When you buy single-serve plastic containers or cans of fruit, look for unsweetened fruit packed in water instead of light or heavy syrup, or candied.
- Dried fruit. Look for dried fruit that's unsweetened.
- 100% fruit juice. Buy juices that say 100% fruit juice on the label (for example, orange juice, apple juice, cranberry juice, and grape juice); otherwise, you're likely getting extra sugar and calories without the full range of nutrients that 100% fruit juices can provide.

Vegetables

When you buy vegetables (including nonstarchy, starchy, and legumes), make sure to look for those in their lowest sugar, lowest fat form. Following are some additional tips to help you make more healthful vegetable selections:

Fresh and frozen vegetables: Choose a variety of colorful vegetables, starchy and nonstarchy, that are prepared without any added fats (such as butter or cream sauce), breading (for example, breaded onion rings), added sugars, or added salt. Here are some vegetables that are loaded with fiber, vitamins, minerals, and antioxidants:

- Fiber—artichokes, brussels sprouts, baby carrots, chiles (hot peppers), jicamas, frozen mixed vegetables (corn, green beans, and carrots, or lima beans and corn), peas, pumpkin, winter squash, and sweet potatoes; among the legumes, pinto beans, chickpeas, kidney beans, navy beans, northern beans, and soybeans pack in the most fiber.
- Vitamin A—carrots, sweet potatoes, pumpkin, spinach, collards, and turnip greens.
- Vitamin C—broccoli, peppers, tomatoes, cabbage, potatoes, romaine lettuce, turnip greens, and spinach.
- Folate—cooked dried beans and peas, spinach, and mustard greens.
- Potassium—baked white or sweet potatoes, cooked greens (such as spinach), and winter squash.
- Antioxidants—small red beans, red kidney beans, pinto beans, and black beans.

Canned vegetables: When you buy canned vegetables, look for those that are not creamed, candied, pickled, or made with syrup (these add sugar and calories); pickles are generally high in added sugars as well.

100% vegetable juice: If you or your kids like the taste of vegetable juice, look for low-sodium varieties (those with 140 milligrams or less per serving).

Grains

When you're shopping for grains (hot or cold cereal, breads, pasta, rice, and crackers), look first for whole-grain selections. It can be quite confusing to find whole-grain foods. The best way is to take a look at the ingredients list on the food package. You cannot rely on the color of foods (for example, brown bread) or descriptive names such as "multigrain," "seven-grain," or "cracked wheat" to find whole grains. The only way really to know if what you're consuming is a whole grain is to check out the ingredients list on the food package. A whole-grain food is one in which the first ingredient listed is a whole grain—the words *whole* or *whole grain* before the grain ingredient's name will be listed first on the ingredients list. Examples include whole wheat, whole oat, whole-grain corn, and whole rye. Other whole grains include barley, buckwheat, bulgur, brown rice, millet, popcorn, rye, sorghum, and wild rice.

Because whole grains offer up so many health benefits, make most of your cereal, bread, pasta, and rice selections whole grain. Following are some other things to look for on food labels when you and your family are shopping for grains:

When You Buy:	Look For:
Breads or crackers	A whole grain listed as the first ingredient, 3 grams or less of fat; no saturated fat or trans fats; at least 3 to 5 grams of fiber per serving; no added sugar
Hot or cold cereals	A whole grain listed as the first ingredient; 3 grams or less of fat; no saturated fat or trans fats; at least 3 to 5 grams of fiber per serving; less than 10 grams of added sugar
Pasta or rice	A whole grain listed as the first ingredient
Frozen waffles or pancakes	A whole grain listed as the first ingredient; 3 grams or less of fat; no saturated fat or trans fats; at least 3 to 5 grams of fiber per serving; and less than 5 grams of sugar

Although you want half of your grains to come from whole grains, you can incorporate some refined grains such as waffles or French bread into your diet; when you opt for refined grains, the fiber content will likely be lower. If you choose some refined foods, make sure to choose other high-fiber grain, fruit, and/or vegetable selections that day to meet your individual fiber needs (see appendix D).

Snacks Disguised as Grains

Many snack foods, including breakfast bars, energy bars, cereal bars, granola bars, pretzels, popcorn, and chips, are, in part, counted as grains. But because many of these foods are loaded with any combination of calories, fat, and sugar, and few are actually whole grains, it's best to count these foods as extra calories. Of course there are always exceptions, and if you read enough food labels you may actually find a healthy snack offering from among these items. As a good rule of thumb, when you do choose these foods, look for those that have 3 grams of fat or less and no saturated or trans fats (see the box "How to Avoid Trans-Fat Traps" on this page) and less than 8 grams of sugar; also, opt for foods that are baked and not fried to minimize any damage to your heart or your waistline.

How to Avoid Trans-Fat Traps

Here are some quick label-reading tips to help you and your family curb your trans fat intake without driving yourselves crazy:

- Look for 0 grams of trans fats on food labels. But be aware that a product that contains trans fats—but less than 0.5 grams per serving—can say it has 0 grams.

- Read the ingredients list; if you find the words *partially hydrogenated*, then the product does contain some trans fats. Look for an alternative food without these ingredients. If you do choose to have foods that list trans fats in the ingredients list, be sure to stick to one serving. Because many products that contain trans fats are snack foods that a lot of us (not just the kids) tend to overdo, having two or more servings can really increase your trans fat intake.

- Many foods high in trans fats are also high in saturated fat. Stick to less than 10 percent of your total calorie intake from saturated and trans fats combined.

Meats and Beans

Following are some tips to help you and your family make smarter selections when you shop for meat, poultry, fish, legumes, eggs, nuts, and seeds to maximize the nutrients these foods contain and minimize calories, fat, saturated fat, cholesterol, and sodium.

Meat and poultry: Because meats and poultry can pack in calories, fat, saturated fat, and cholesterol, select the leanest cuts. Have more of these lower fat selections:

- Lean cuts of beef (including round eye, top round, bottom round, round tip, top loin, and top sirloin)
- Skinless white meat chicken or turkey breast
- Extralean (at least 90 percent lean) ground round, ground sirloin, ground chicken, or ground turkey
- Lean cuts of pork (including pork loin, tenderloin, center loin, and lean ham),
- Canadian bacon

Have less of these high-fat selections:

- Cold cuts and lunch meats
- Hot dogs
- Bacon
- Duck
- Goose
- Some cuts of beef (ground beef, chuck, rib, or brisket)

Many of these selections are also high in sodium, so having less of them can help you curb your sodium intake.

Fish: Fish is a great source of key nutrients, including omega-3 fats (especially fatty fish, such as wild salmon, herring, pollock, flounder or sole, or halibut). Choose any variety of fresh fish or shellfish you enjoy (if you have high cholesterol or heart disease, emphasize fish over shellfish because of the high cholesterol content of shellfish). If you choose frozen fish or frozen meals that include fish, look for those that are not breaded, made with cream, butter, or high-fat sources, or containing trans fats. When you shop for canned fish, look for those packed in water instead of oil, and rinse to lower their sodium content. If you are pregnant, nursing, or a young child, the FDA advises you to choose low-mercury fish options such as shrimp, canned light tuna, salmon, pollock, and catfish and to avoid shark, swordfish, tilefish, and king mackerel.

Legumes: Beans and peas are available in bins for you to choose from yourself, in plastic packages, and in cans. When you buy canned beans, look for low-sodium varieties; baked beans and chili made with beans can also be sources of added sugar, so be sure to read labels.

Eggs: A variety of eggs and egg substitutes are available at the grocery store. To save on calories, saturated fat, and cholesterol, you can buy egg substitutes to use in any recipe that calls for eggs.

Nuts, seeds, and nut butters: Look for nuts and seeds made without added sodium. Because many commercially prepared nut butters contain added sugar, read labels to find sugar-free alternatives. Although all nuts are healthful, they are also high in calories and fat. Here's a comparison for some popular nuts, from least to most:

Type of Nut	Calories (per ounce)
Cashews	157
Pistachio	158
Peanuts	166
Almonds	169
Walnuts	185
Pecans	201
Macadamias	203

Milk, Yogurt, and Cheese

Because milk, yogurt, and cheese, in their full-fat forms, provide substantial amounts of calories, fat, saturated fat, and cholesterol, it's wise to look for low-fat and nonfat options in the dairy aisle for all the members of your family over the age of two. Also, because many foods made with milk (including yogurt, ice cream, and puddings) can be loaded with sugar as well, it's key to read labels and see how much sugar these foods really contain. Following are some tips to help you and your family make healthier selections from the abundance of dairy foods available at your supermarket:

Milk: Choose 1% or skim milk to drink or use to make hot cereals or in recipes; if you choose chocolate milks or any flavored milks, be aware that they can have a lot of added sugar and extra calories. Having one cup of chocolate milk is like having one cup of low-fat milk and a cookie. These milks are likely to have significantly less added sugar than that found in soft drinks and juice drinks, however, so I'd argue they're still a good bet for your kids if they won't drink plain low-fat, or skim milk. Also, a variety of low-fat milks have the thicker texture of 2% or whole milk. These milks can help ease the transition from high-fat milks to low-fat milks as your children grow. When you buy puddings or other foods made with milk, look for those that are low in fat (3 grams of fat or less) and low in added sugar or sugar-free. If you choose full-fat pudding or ice cream, be sure to have small portions and factor in the extra calories. If you or your children can't tolerate milk because of lactose intolerance, look for low-fat lactose-free options.

Yogurt: Choose low-fat and nonfat options as often as possible. Be aware that cup for cup, even low-fat or nonfat yogurt may have a lot more calories than skim or 1% milk. Also, when you buy yogurt, keep in mind that plain yogurt has little added sugar, whereas flavored yogurt, fruited yogurt, and yogurt drinks typically contain a lot of added sugar. But again, they're still packed with calcium and other vital nutrients that can benefit your health.

Cheese: Cheese can be another good way to add some calcium to your diet. However, full-fat cheese can add a lot of calories and saturated fat to meals, especially if the portions you consume are large. Fortunately, a variety of reduced fat and low-fat cheeses are available. There are also many forms of cheese that can help you use less and save some calories and fat. For example, shredded or grated cheese can cover a lot more surface area than a slice of cheese and can make a great addition to soups, salads, pasta dishes, and other items. If you can't bear the thought of low-fat cheese, buy the kinds you like but stick to no more than an ounce or two a day to keep calories and saturated fat in check.

Oils

Foods that fit into the oils category include vegetable oils, trans fat–free soft margarine, mayonnaise, and salad dressings. These all provide fat calories, although the calories come from healthful monounsaturated and polyunsaturated fats (see "Fat Facts" on page 144). To get more mileage without increasing your calorie or fat intake, you can choose from an array of reduced fat and low-fat versions of margarine, mayonnaise, and salad dressings. You can also reduce your intake of all these oils with a variety of condiments including mustard and balsamic vinegar (see the box "All About Condiments" on page 154).

For those times when you want a decent meal but don't feel like cooking, your local grocery store is likely to have a variety of prepared foods to please your palate. See the box "Supermarket Takeout" on page 155 to help you make the most healthful selections.

Sugar by Any Other Name Is Just as Sweet and High Calorie

If you're looking to avoid or limit the amount of sugar you and your family consume, one way to do this is by reading food labels. Sugar is listed on ingredient lists under a variety of aliases (see the box "Hidden Sugars" on this page). Although overconsumption of calories from many sources plays a key role in obesity, one sweetener that has been blamed for Americans' expanding waistlines is high fructose corn syrup (HFCS), a sweetener composed of 55 percent fructose and 45 percent glucose. Because it's cheap to produce and adds shelf life to foods, it's added to a variety of high-calorie, low-nutrient foods including packaged snacks and soft drinks. HFCS, like all sugars, is often found in foods and beverages

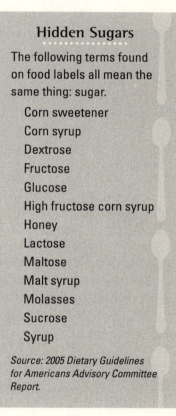

Hidden Sugars

The following terms found on food labels all mean the same thing: sugar.

Corn sweetener

Corn syrup

Dextrose

Fructose

Glucose

High fructose corn syrup

Honey

Lactose

Maltose

Malt syrup

Molasses

Sucrose

Syrup

Source: 2005 Dietary Guidelines for Americans Advisory Committee Report.

that offer little nutritional value to begin with, so it's wise to limit your intake of all foods that contain added sugars including HFCS.

The World Health Organization recommends that no more than 10 percent of daily calories come from "free" sugar (that's the sugar added to food and the concentrated sugars found in fruit juice). For someone who consumes 2,000 calories a day, that's 200 calories, or 40 grams of sugar per day.

All About Condiments

Fortunately, a variety of condiments are low in calories and packed with nutrients to promote health and fight disease. Because many of us, especially kids, love to dip things, condiments are a great way to encourage the family to down those carrot, celery, and bell pepper strips, not to mention whole-grain crackers. Just remember, when it comes to condiments, a little goes a long way. Keep the serving small (up to 2 or 3 tablespoons). The following will add great flavor and texture to any meal and are a great alternative to condiments that are higher in calories, fat, and/or sodium.

- Chutney—has about 25 calories per tablespoon and about 1 gram of fat. It also contains fiber that can fill you up. It can be made with fruits such as apricots (loaded with beta-carotene) or cranberries (high in anthocyanins, plant substances that have antioxidant and anticancer properties and other health benefits), and it tastes great with fish or as a sandwich topping.

- Salsa—has only 7.5 calories per tablespoon. It typically is made with tomatoes (high in lycopene) and onions (which contain the antioxidant quercetin, also found in tea and apples) that help protect the body's cells against free radical damage. (Be sure to look for low-sodium salsa because otherwise it can pack in 85 milligrams per tablespoon).

- Hummus—has about 25 calories and 1.5 grams of fat per tablespoon. It is made from chickpeas (garbanzo beans), it makes a great low-fat protein source, and it also contains soluble fiber that aids digestion and keeps cholesterol levels down.

- Guacamole—has about 15 calories and 1 gram of fat per tablespoon. It is made from avocado, which is high in monounsaturated fat, the kind that promotes heart health and helps keep cholesterol levels down. Avocados also contain fiber, potassium, and folic acid.

- Prepared yellow mustard and horseradish—have less than 10 calories per tablespoon. They both contain zeaxanthin, an antioxidant thought to enhance immune function.

Supermarket Takeout

Tempted by supermarket takeout? A vast array of ready-to-eat meals from wokeries, wood-burning ovens, and sushi bars, and ready-to-cook foods like marinated meats and vegetables are increasingly offered at supermarkets and specialty food markets across the country to provide time-starved families with delicious meals that save them valuable kitchen time. Some offerings may resemble the healthful meals you prepare at home, but others can be more like your usual restaurant fare and are loaded with calories, fat, and sodium. Use these tips before you feast on supermarket takeout:

- Choose foods that are baked, broiled, grilled, or lightly sauteed instead of fried.
- When you buy meats, poultry, or fish, look for those made with or marinated with low-fat, low-calorie condiments like salsa, chutney, Dijon mustard, whole-grain mustard, balsamic vinegar, or horseradish instead of creamy sauces, sour cream, butter, or a lot of oil.
- Instead of meat or poultry dishes, opt for baked fish or other protein-rich foods that you may not make too often (or ever) at home, including edamame, tempeh, or tabouleh.
- As a substitute for run-of-the-mill rice or pasta, tempt your family with some grains you don't make at home, such as amaranth, quinoa, or wheat berries.

As you can see, it is well worth taking the time to read labels carefully in the supermarket to help you and your family make better, more informed food choices.

The Ultimate Family Food Shopping List

On the following pages you will find a comprehensive list of a variety of items (including those that are found in the two weeks of delicious meal plans in chapter 14). There are spaces in each category for you to write in additional items you and your family enjoy. Before you use this list, think about what you'll need for the upcoming week to feed yourself and your family. Copy this list and place it on your refrigerator door or kitchen bulletin board as a reminder of what to buy each week.

FRUITS

Fresh Fruit (or packaged fresh):

- ❏ Apples—green, red
- ❏ Avocado
- ❏ Bananas
- ❏ Blueberries
- ❏ Cantaloupes
- ❏ Clementines
- ❏ Honeydew melons
- ❏ Kiwifruits
- ❏ Lemons
- ❏ Mandarin oranges
- ❏ Mangoes

- ❏ Oranges
- ❏ Peaches
- ❏ Pears
- ❏ Plums
- ❏ Raspberries
- ❏ Red grapes
- ❏ Strawberries
- ❏ _____
- ❏ _____
- ❏ _____
- ❏ _____

Canned, Jarred Fruit, or Fruit in Snack Packs (without added sugar):

- ❏ Natural applesauce
- ❏ Pineapple chunks, canned in water

- ❏ _____
- ❏ _____
- ❏ _____

Frozen Fruits (without added sugar):

- ❏ _____
- ❏ _____

- ❏ _____
- ❏ _____

Dried Fruit (without added sugar):

- ❏ Dried fruit bits
- ❏ Golden raisins
- ❏ Raisins
- ❏ _____

- ❏ _____
- ❏ _____
- ❏ _____

100% Fruit Juices:

- ❏ Lime juice
- ❏ Orange juice

- ❏ _____
- ❏ _____

Other:

- ❏ _____
- ❏ _____

- ❏ _____
- ❏ _____

VEGETABLES

Fresh Vegetables (or packaged fresh):

- ❏ Arugula
- ❏ Asparagus
- ❏ Broccoli
- ❏ Broccoli rabe
- ❏ Brussels sprouts
- ❏ Cabbage, shredded
- ❏ Carrots, whole, baby, and shredded
- ❏ Celery
- ❏ Cucumbers
- ❏ Endive
- ❏ Eggplant
- ❏ Green beans
- ❏ Jalapeño peppers
- ❏ Mixed green salad leaves
- ❏ Mushrooms—shiitake, portobello

- ❏ Onions—red and white
- ❏ Peppers—green, red, and yellow
- ❏ Potatoes
- ❏ Romaine lettuce
- ❏ Scallions
- ❏ Squash, butternut (winter)
- ❏ Sweet potatoes
- ❏ Tomatoes—cherry, plum, and red
- ❏ Zucchini
- ❏ _____
- ❏ _____
- ❏ _____
- ❏ _____
- ❏ _____
- ❏ _____

Canned or Jarred Vegetables (make most choices low sodium or no salt added and no sugar added):

- ❏ Corn
- ❏ Peas and carrots
- ❏ Pumpkin, purée
- ❏ Salsa
- ❏ Tomatoes, plum, peeled
- ❏ Tomato paste

- ❏ Tomato sauce, low-sodium
- ❏ _____
- ❏ _____
- ❏ _____
- ❏ _____

Frozen Vegetables (without added fats):

- ❏ Broccoli florets
- ❏ Spinach, chopped

- ❏ _____
- ❏ _____

BEANS/LEGUMES

- ❑ Black beans, canned (low sodium or no salt added)
- ❑ Garbanzo beans (chickpeas) (low sodium or no salt added)
- ❑ Kidney beans, canned (low sodium or no salt added)
- ❑ Lentils
- ❑ Refried beans
- ❑ Soy crumbles
- ❑ Tofu, extra firm, made with calcium
- ❑ Vegetarian refried beans
- ❑ _____
- ❑ _____
- ❑ _____
- ❑ _____

GRAINS

Breads and Bread Products:

- ❑ Flour tortillas—whole-wheat and white
- ❑ Italian bread
- ❑ Whole-grain waffles
- ❑ Whole-wheat bread
- ❑ Whole-wheat English muffins
- ❑ Whole-wheat pita
- ❑ Whole-wheat sub rolls
- ❑ _____
- ❑ _____
- ❑ _____
- ❑ _____

Cereals:

- ❑ Bran flakes
- ❑ Corn flakes
- ❑ Granola cereal, low fat (no added raisins)
- ❑ Kellogg's Special K cereal
- ❑ Multigrain Cheerios
- ❑ Oat bran flakes
- ❑ Oatmeal
- ❑ Oats, rolled
- ❑ _____
- ❑ _____
- ❑ _____

Crackers:

- ❑ Graham crackers
- ❑ Whole-wheat crackers
- ❑ _____
- ❑ _____
- ❑ _____

Rice:

- ❏ Brown rice
- ❏ Wild rice
- ❏ _____

- ❏ _____
- ❏ _____

Pasta:

- ❏ Elbow macaroni—whole wheat
- ❏ Fusilli
- ❏ Lasagna noodles
- ❏ Linguini—whole wheat

- ❏ Penne—whole wheat
- ❏ Spaghetti
- ❏ _____
- ❏ _____
- ❏ _____

Other Grains:

- ❏ Bread crumbs
- ❏ Couscous
- ❏ Croutons, fat free
- ❏ Flour—white, whole wheat
- ❏ Ginger snaps
- ❏ Pancake and waffle mix, complete
- ❏ Popcorn (unsalted, bagged, or kernels)

- ❏ Pretzels
- ❏ Tortilla chips, baked
- ❏ Wheat germ
- ❏ Whole-wheat pretzels
- ❏ _____
- ❏ _____
- ❏ _____

MILK/YOGURT/CHEESE

Milk:

- ❏ Buttermilk, low fat (1%)
- ❏ Evaporated milk, fat free
- ❏ Milk, skim
- ❏ Milk, low fat (1%)

- ❏ _____
- ❏ _____
- ❏ _____

Yogurt:

- ❏ Nonfat yogurt, vanilla
- ❏ Low-fat yogurt, plain
- ❏ Low-fat yogurt, vanilla

- ❏ _____
- ❏ _____
- ❏ _____

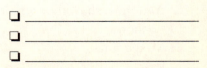

Cheese (natural or processed):

- ❏ American cheese
- ❏ Cheddar cheese, reduced fat or low fat, shredded
- ❏ Cottage cheese, low fat
- ❏ Mozzarella cheese, low moisture, part skim

- ❏ Parmesan cheese, grated
- ❏ Ricotta cheese, low fat
- ❏ Swiss cheese
- ❏ _____
- ❏ _____
- ❏ _____

Other:

- ❏ Ice cream, vanilla (or any flavor)
- ❏ Pudding cups, chocolate/vanilla swirl or any flavor

- ❏ _____
- ❏ _____
- ❏ _____

BEEF/POULTRY/FISH

Beef/Poultry:

- ❏ Chicken breast, boneless, skinless
- ❏ Chicken breast, lean, ground
- ❏ Chicken, drumsticks, skinless
- ❏ Chicken or turkey sausage

- ❏ Pork chops
- ❏ Sirloin steak
- ❏ Turkey, fresh roasted
- ❏ Turkey breast, lean, ground
- ❏ _____
- ❏ _____
- ❏ _____

Fish:

- ❏ Cod filets
- ❏ Salmon filets
- ❏ Shrimp, large
- ❏ Tuna, light, canned, packed in water

- ❏ _____
- ❏ _____
- ❏ _____

NUTS/NUT BUTTERS/SEEDS (unsalted)

- ❏ Almonds, shaved or whole
- ❏ Cashews
- ❏ Mixed nuts
- ❏ Peanut butter, natural (no added sugar)

- ❏ Walnut halves
- ❏ _____
- ❏ _____
- ❏ _____

EGGS

- ❑ Large eggs
- ❑ Egg substitute
- ❑ _____
- ❑ _____
- ❑ _____

OILS

- ❑ Balsamic vinaigrette salad dressing
- ❑ Canola oil
- ❑ Creamy Italian salad dressing
- ❑ Italian salad dressing
- ❑ Margarine, soft tub, with no trans fats
- ❑ Mayonnaise
- ❑ Olive oil
- ❑ Olive oil spray
- ❑ Ranch dressing, reduced fat
- ❑ _____
- ❑ _____
- ❑ _____

CONDIMENTS/HERBS/SPICES/SEASONINGS
(low-sodium versions, if possible):

- ❑ Balsamic vinegar
- ❑ Basil
- ❑ Bay leaf
- ❑ Black pepper, ground
- ❑ Chili powder
- ❑ Chili seasoning mix, low sodium
- ❑ Chipotle pepper
- ❑ Cilantro
- ❑ Clove (ground)
- ❑ Coriander
- ❑ Cumin
- ❑ Curry powder
- ❑ Cinnamon
- ❑ Dill
- ❑ Garlic—cloves, powder
- ❑ Ginger—chopped, crystallized
- ❑ Ketchup
- ❑ Kosher salt
- ❑ Mint
- ❑ Mustard, whole grain
- ❑ Nutmeg
- ❑ Onion powder
- ❑ Oregano
- ❑ Paprika
- ❑ Parsley
- ❑ Red pepper flakes, crushed
- ❑ Rosemary
- ❑ Sage
- ❑ Salt
- ❑ Sea salt
- ❑ Southwestern seasoning blend (like Emeril's)
- ❑ Soy sauce, low sodium
- ❑ Tabasco chipotle pepper sauce
- ❑ Thyme

CONDIMENTS/HERBS/SPICES/SEASONINGS (*continued*)

- ❏ Tarragon leaves, dried
- ❏ Teriyaki sauce, light
- ❏ Worcestershire sauce

- ❏ _____
- ❏ _____
- ❏ _____

OTHER FOODS (solid fats, sugary foods or foods with added sugars, alcoholic beverages, baking items, miscellaneous):

- ❏ Brown sugar
- ❏ Coconut, shredded
- ❏ Chicken broth, low sodium
- ❏ Chocolate, dark
- ❏ Chocolate chips, semisweet or milk
- ❏ Chocolate chip cookies
- ❏ Cocoa powder
- ❏ Coconut extract
- ❏ Coconut, shredded
- ❏ Cream cheese (Neufchâtel)

- ❏ Maple syrup, light
- ❏ Nonstick cooking spray
- ❏ Sour cream, reduced fat or nonfat
- ❏ Spanish sherry
- ❏ Sugar—cane, powdered
- ❏ Sugar—brown
- ❏ Vanilla extract
- ❏ _____
- ❏ _____
- ❏ _____

BEVERAGES

- ❏ Coffee
- ❏ Iced tea, unsweetened
- ❏ Water, carbonated
- ❏ Water, bottled

- ❏ _____
- ❏ _____
- ❏ _____

MISCELLANEOUS

- ❏ _____
- ❏ _____

- ❏ _____
- ❏ _____

13

Eating Out While Still Eating Healthfully

If your family is like most, you get more and more of your calories away from home. Whether you eat at a fast-food or sit-down restaurant, have dinner at a ball game or the circus, grab a snack from a vending machine, convenience store, or local coffee bar, or you're at a party or some sort of social gathering, chances are you're taking in more calories than you need to maintain a healthy body weight. Not only are portions at these places huge, but the more food you're offered, the more calories you're likely to consume. Also, because we are constantly bombarded with ads for highly palatable foods and beverages that are high in calories, fat, and/or sugar on TV and billboards, and then we see and smell these foods just about wherever we go, twenty-four hours a day, seven days a week, it's not surprising that most of us have a tough time making healthful selections and keeping tabs on how much we consume when we venture out to eat.

The good news is that no matter how often you and your family eat out or get your sustenance when you're away from home, you can all learn how to plan ahead and be better prepared to make more healthful selections to help you meet your individual nutrient needs and maintain a healthy weight.

The Portion Problem

Eating out is a challenge because usually we're offered larger portions than we would serve ourselves at home. Also, although nutrition information for menu items may be available at some restaurants, many times we're left in the dark about calories, fat grams, and other nutritional information when we eat out. That's why it's critical, especially if you and your family eat out often, to get a good sense of what realistic portions for you look like (see appendix E for a chart that helps you eyeball portion sizes when you eat out). Having large portions regularly can lead to excess calorie consumption that can eventually cause weight gain, so the number-one rule when eating on-the-go is: no matter what foods you choose, keep portions small to reduce the chances you'll consume more calories than your body can use.

Fitting in Fast Food

I admit I have many fast-food memories. I still remember going to Burger King for lunch with my mom on my fourth birthday. The crown, the burger, and the fries—what more could a four-year-old ask for? How about the time my Nana drove to my sleepaway camp to deliver my favorite indulgence, a BK Whopper with cheese and French fries? My best friend, Mindy, and I devoured it secretly as we sat on a small patch of grass near the dirt road entrance to our camp. And I'll admit that I was quite upset—my mom says I even cried, although I don't remember that—when I found out that the Wendy's near us was going to close down. I grew up with fast food, and my own family indulges in it every once in a while.

We know fast food does not equal healthy food. But the truth is, fast food is a part of many people's lives, not just in the United States but worldwide, and there are no signs it's going away anytime soon. Fast food can fit into an otherwise healthful, nutritious diet, but if you and your family frequent fast-food restaurants often (more than once a week), there's a good chance you're getting more calories, fat, saturated fat and trans fat than you bargained for. But you can make more healthful selections when you opt for fast food. Here are some tips to help you fit in fast food:

- **Plan for fast-food meals.** As a general rule, try not to opt for fast food just because it's convenient for you; plan for it as you would a visit to a sit-down restaurant. For example, you can plan for it when you travel with your family or if you know your family's schedule will be especially hectic one day. If you long for your favorite meal (one that doesn't include whole grains, fruits, or vegetables), make sure to incorporate these healthful foods at other meals that day, and cut back on sugar and added fats to stay within your daily calorie goals (see chapter 10 to determine your individual calorie needs).

- **Get the facts.** Many fast-food establishments—among them, McDonald's, Burger King, Wendy's, KFC, and other chains—provide information about the nutritional content of their items either at the store (perhaps hung on a wall or in a small booklet or flier), on their Web site or even on the items themselves (for example, McDonald's now posts nutrition information on the wrappers or cartons in which foods are served). Learning how many calories and other nutrients are in your favorite foods relative to your estimated daily needs can help you put your fast-food meals in perspective.

- **Buy items à la carte.** Instead of ordering your usual cost-cutting combo meal, ask for individual items only. That way you can better control how many different foods you consume, as well as the portion sizes of each.

- **Go for veggies.** Whether you choose a premade salad or make your own salad at the salad bar, order some type of vegetable that can help you meet your daily quota and fill you up.

- **Downsize.** If you can't resist your usual burger and fries, ask for smaller versions. Even making minor adjustments—getting a small order of French fries instead of a medium order—can save you about 130 calories and 7 grams of fat; if you switch from a large order to a small order, you'll save about 320 calories and about 17 grams of fat.

- **Be choosy about beverages.** When your kids order the kid's meals (no doubt to get the toy inside), encourage them to skip sugary soda and instead ask for low-fat milk. If your child insists on soda, consider it a special treat; let them know that it can be an alternative to cookies or other sweets that day.

- **Keep an eye on add-ons.** Always ask for sandwiches without ketchup, mayonnaise, or special sauce; if you want these condiments, ask for them on the side (fast-food restaurants do usually offer low-fat mayonnaises and salad dressings as options). If a sandwich comes with cheese, ask for only one slice to save fat and calories. Mustard is a great low-calorie option, but limit the amounts because it can be high in sodium.

The Breakfast Club

If you and your family venture out for breakfast or brunch on weekends or on vacation, you can eat out and still eat well. If you're choosing foods from a buffet, take a lap around the food displays to see what your options are before you dive in. Then make it a rule to make only one trip and fill only one plate. After the meal, fill up with water or seltzer, plain or splashed with orange or cranberry juice, or low-fat milk. If you order from a menu, be sure to ask what exactly comes with your meal. For example, if you are hungry for an omelet, you may order one with whole-wheat toast, but may end up getting hash browns and muffins as well. Ask for exactly what you want and ideally, the restaurant will oblige. If there's more on your plate than you bargained for, you can kindly ask the server to remove the extras before you dig in and the temptation overwhelms you. Alternatively, you can order one meal for two and share with a family member—a great idea because the portions served are usually huge. You can use the visuals in appendix E to estimate how much you're actually eating when you grab food on the go.

Following are some healthful breakfast options (portions will vary depending on your individual calorie needs; see chapter 10):

- Egg-white omelet (or scrambled eggs) made with Swiss cheese, mushrooms, peppers, tomatoes, or any other vegetable you choose, served with whole-grain toast with low-sugar jelly or trans fat–free margarine and skim milk
- Fresh fruit salad mixed with low-fat yogurt and whole-wheat toast with trans fat–free margarine
- Oatmeal topped with pecans or walnuts, cinnamon, or brown sugar, and a cup of orange juice

- Bran muffin, served with a cup of low-fat yogurt topped with fresh berries
- French toast made with whole-wheat bread, and a cup of skim milk
- Whole-wheat pancakes or waffles topped with sliced strawberries, bananas, or fresh berries
- Whole-wheat English muffin topped with Canadian bacon and a slice of cheese, and a cup of skim milk
- Whole-wheat bagel with smoked salmon and tomatoes and 1 to 2 teaspoons of cream cheese
- Fresh fruit plate with low-fat cottage cheese and a toasted whole-wheat English muffin

Dining Out Tips for Every Occasion

Many families also celebrate (or simply take a break from takeout or home cooking) by going out for lunch or dinner over the weekend. Because eating out may be a special treat, you certainly don't want to sacrifice good taste or be concerned about every morsel that passes your lips. You want to enjoy your food and have a good time. If you don't want to give up your favorite dishes, have them, just have less. If you eat three quarters of what you normally would, you'll instantly curb your calorie intake. Another good way to save calories is to *eat* most of them. Instead of wasting calories on drinks such as sugary soda, fruit drinks, or alcoholic beverages, why not choose water or seltzer with lemon or lime (or a splash of orange or cranberry juice), unsweetened iced tea, or diet soda? Maybe you cannot bear the thought of giving up that glass of wine or beer, but try to stick to just one, because the calories really add up (see the table on page 168); interestingly, a recent survey by the NPD Group found that adults who drank wine with their meals were more likely to order dessert than those who did not consume wine.

Perhaps you can allow your kids to have one small cup or glass of soda or a fruity drink if they really want one, as a special treat when you go out for dinner instead of keeping such beverages at home. On vacations, when the family eats out constantly, the rule can be one soda a day or every other day.

Calorie Counts for Alcohol		
Beverage	**Amount (in ounces)**	**Approximate Total Calories***
Beer (regular)	12	144
Beer (light)	12	108
White wine	5	100
Red wine	5	105
Sweet dessert wine	3	141
80 proof distilled spirits (gin, rum, vodka, whiskey)	1.5	96

Source: USDA, Dietary Guidelines for Americans 2005, 6th Ed.
*The total calories and alcohol content vary depending on the brand. Moreover, adding mixers to an alcoholic beverage can contribute calories in addition to the calories from the alcohol itself.

No matter what type of cuisine you choose, here are some suggestions to help you and your family navigate through your next meal out:

When you order:
- Ask for what you want, and teach your kids to do the same (politely, of course).
- Ask questions if you don't understand all the terms on the menu; ask how dishes are prepared and ask what comes on the side.
- Order dishes prepared in a healthful way: broiled, baked, steamed, roasted, poached, dry broiled (in wine or lemon juice), stir-fried, or lightly sautéed instead of breaded, fried, or prepared in a creamy, buttery, or oily sauce. For kids' dishes, you (or your kids) can ask for grilled cheese made with whole-wheat bread instead of white bread or have pasta served with tomato sauce or olive oil on the side instead of drowned in butter or cheese sauce.
- Ask for substitutions. For example, if you already had bread or chips, skip the starch and ask for a vegetable instead; if your dish comes with fried vegetables, ask for grilled or steamed vegetables instead. Even kids can request fruit salad or apple sauce as alternatives to French fries.
- If you want an appetizer, start with grilled, steamed, or lightly sautéed vegetables, broth- or vegetable-based soups, or a colorful salad with dressing on the side. These can fill you up and prevent you from overeating when your entrée arrives.
- Order all sauces, salad dressings, condiments, and other toppings on the side.

- Share appetizers, order half-orders of pasta, and share entrées with other family members.
- Because kids' menus are usually loaded with fried, greasy, high-fat foods such as creamy macaroni and cheese, burgers, hot dogs, grilled cheese, pasta with butter, and French fries and other fried foods, you may want to forgo the children's menu completely and share your own meal with one of your children. If your kids are used to ordering "kid food," encourage them to order for themselves and make more healthful selections and substitutions (as suggested here). You can also order extra vegetables or share yours to supplement their meals.

When you eat:
- Ask your waiter to remove the bread or chip basket from the table once you (and others at your table) have had enough. Alternatively, you can bypass it entirely to save room for appetizers and entrées.
- Eat slowly and enjoy each bite; put your fork down between bites. Although it's not always easy to focus on your food when you're also feeding your kids (especially young ones), try to make mealtimes pleasant.
- If you're feeling full but there's still food on your plate, ask the waiter to wrap it up on ice; that way you will resist the temptation to continue eating if the food remains right in front of you.
- If dessert is a must, this can be a great time to meet your fruit quota with fresh berries or sliced fruit; sherbet or biscotti are also low-calorie, low-fat alternatives to cakes and pies. Make it a rule to share your dessert with your family, and be sure to savor each bite. If you insist on your own dessert, it's still a good idea to share because portions tend to be huge; just be sure to save up your extra calories (see page 113) to splurge on dessert instead of having them during the day.

Drowning in Coffee

In recent years, coffee bars have become a top hangout spot, for both adults and children. Even older children and teens flock to coffee bars after school or on weekends and feast on decadent coffee beverages in oversized cups. Caffeine, a central nervous system stimulant, can have pronounced effects in children; avoid offering caffeinated beverages such as coffee, soft drinks, and energy drinks, especially because many of the drinks that contain caffeine are also loaded with artificial sweeteners, calories, sugar, and/or fat. Basic black coffee provides less than 10 calories for 16 ounces (a typical serving size), but many coffee beverages pack in 400 or 500 calories because they're made with whole milk, sugar, and other add-ons. Here are some tips to help you skim the calories and fat from your coffee:

- **Decrease your cup size.** Switching from a 16-ounce cup to a 10- or 12-ounce cup can help you slash calories but still enjoy the taste of your coffee.

- **Skim your milk.** If your favorite coffee is made with whole milk, ask for low-fat (1%) or skim milk instead to save calories and harmful saturated fat.

- **Use low-calorie add-ons.** Skip the whipped cream (which provides 60 calories and 6 grams of fat for 2 tablespoons) and half-and-half (40 calories for 2 tablespoons) and opt instead for fat-free half-and-half (20 calories for 2 tablespoons), sugar (11 calories per packet), or a packet of an artificial sweetener (0 calories) to sweeten your coffee.

- **Make substitutions.** Instead of coffee, opt for low-calorie cappuccino, espresso, or tea as an alternative once in a while.

- **Save it for a special occasion.** If you must have your decadent coffee beverage, save it for a once- or twice-weekly treat instead of a daily indulgence.

Temptations of the Feast

Because it's likely that the sight and smell of food—oh, so glorious food—at birthday parties, cocktail parties, school events, weddings, family get-togethers, and family outings (the circus or a ball game) can overwhelm you and lead you and your family to overeat, try to anticipate as much as possible what you'll eat, and plan the rest of your menu selections that day accordingly. If the food is served buffet style, following are a few tips to help you and your family make better selections that won't derail your healthy eating efforts:

- If you're going to an event where you know the food will be tempting, plan ahead. During that day, and for a few days before, try to limit the extra calories you consume—for example, skip your nightly ice cream ritual or that midday piece of chocolate; also go easy on your oils and other added fats because they add a lot of calories in a small quantity (for example, you can use mustard instead of mayonnaise in sandwiches, scramble your eggs with nonstick cooking spray, or top your whole-grain toast with low-sugar jelly instead of margarine). All these small savings in calories can add up over the week so you can afford some extra calories at the event itself.

- Instead of skipping a meal to save calories (which can lead to extreme hunger that can set you up to overeat), have your usual meal in a smaller portion and plan to have a snack high in fiber and protein to fill you up and curb hunger. Some examples include cheese and whole-grain crackers, homemade trail mix with nuts, dried fruit, and crunchy whole-grain cereal, or a low-fat yogurt topped with berries.

- If you're at a buffet-style event, before you stand on line and mindlessly fill your plate, take a lap to see what's available. Make only one trip to the buffet and have only enough food to fit on one plate. Fill half your plate with colorful vegetables such as salad greens or grilled vegetables or fruit, fill a quarter with some sort of lean protein, such as sliced turkey, grilled chicken, fish, lean roast beef, beans, and/or cheese; and use the other quarter of your plate for a starchy vegetable such as potatoes or a grain such as rice, couscous, or pasta (but make sure these foods are not drowned in oil).

- Fill up on low-calorie or calorie-free beverages including water, seltzer, and unsweetened iced tea instead of sugary soda or alcohol. Try to limit liquid calories to just one drink (for adults, that can be one glass of wine or 12 ounces of beer, and for kids, that can be one cup of apple juice or the can of soda they save for when they go out). Keep in mind that caloric drinks provide a lot of calories but won't fill you up the way food does, and too much alcohol can lead you to eat more.

Most of all, remember to have fun! You can certainly enjoy the food, but it's also a great time to focus more on friends and family and enjoy the company.

As you can see, it's tough but not impossible to make healthier selections whether you and your family eat at or grab take-out from a fast-food or sit-down restaurant (or even from your local supermarket, which is likely well stocked with freshly made heat-and-eat meals), or go to an event or social gathering. With the tips in this book, you and your family can make more mindful selections and better control your portions to support your individual nutrient needs and weight management efforts.

14

Delicious Meal Plans

In this chapter you'll find two weeks of carefully crafted menus to help you and your family members above the age of two eat in a way that's more consistent with the Ultimate Family Food Guide in chapter 10. On average, each daily menu plan provides approximately 1,600 calories, the estimated calorie needs for many children, older women, or women who want to lose weight. It incorporates at minimum the amounts recommended for each food group based on that calorie pattern (see page 96 and chapter 10 to determine the number of calories and accompanying food pattern that's right for you and other family members based on age, stage of life, and individual weight goals).

These menus are also consistent with the recommendations made by the Dietary Guidelines for Americans, and on average, they provide 20 to 35 percent calories from total fat, less than 10 percent calories from saturated fat, less than 300 milligrams of dietary cholesterol, and less than 2,300 milligrams of sodium. They are also low in trans fats and added sugars, and provide adequate fiber (see appendix D to determine your individual fiber needs). On each daily menu, you will see items marked with an asterisk; these indicate many of the family-friendly recipes that can be found in chapter 15.

In addition, these menus are filled with a variety of the most nutrient-dense foods (vegetables, fruits, whole grains, nuts, and fish) as well as small amounts of foods that would otherwise be off-limits (especially if weight loss is your goal), such as cookies and sausage. No food is a no-no, and these menus illustrate that you don't need to deprive yourself or avoid certain foods to manage your weight. You can actually consume a diet filled with nutritious and delicious foods (and small amounts of indulgences) in sensible proportions.

As you look through the two weeks of menus, you'll find a variety of breakfasts, lunches, dinners, and snacks and desserts. Next to each item, you'll find in parentheses what it counts as in terms of the food categories illustrated in the "Ultimate Family Food Guide" (see chapter 10). If your daily meal pattern calls for 1,600 calories, you can follow these menu plans as is or adapt some or all of them with alternative items from each food category found in the "Master Food Lists" in appendix G. To adapt the menu to meet the needs of a family member who follows a 1,200-calorie meal pattern (for a four- or five-year-old child, for example), you can subtract the following from the daily menu:

½ cup fruit

½ cup vegetable

1 grain

2 meats

1 milk

1½ teaspoons oil

Alternatively, to adapt the menu upward to meet the needs of a family member who wants to consume a 2,000-calorie meal pattern (for example, an older boy or a man), you can add the following items to the current menu:

½ cup fruit

½ cup vegetable

1 grain

½ meat/beans

1 oil

Day 1

Breakfast

  2 whole-grain waffles (2 grains)
  2 tablespoons light pancake syrup (50 extra calories)
  ½ cup sliced strawberries (½ cup fruit)
  1 cup skim milk (1 milk/yogurt/cheese)
  2 teaspoons trans fat–free margarine (2 oils)

Lunch

  Salad made with:
     3 ounces grilled chicken breast, cut in strips (3 meat/beans)
     ¼ cup garbanzo beans (1 meat/beans)
     2 cups romaine lettuce (1 cup vegetables)
     ½ cup red and yellow pepper strips (½ cup vegetables)
     2 tablespoons creamy Italian salad dressing (2 oils)
  1 slice whole-wheat bread (1 grain)

Dinner

  Extra Creamy Macaroni and Cheese* (2 grains plus 1¼ milk/yogurt/cheese)
  ½ cup baby carrots (½ cup vegetables)

Snacks/Desserts

  1 cup (8 ounces) low-fat yogurt, plain (1 milk/yogurt/cheese)
  1 cup blueberries (1 cup fruit)
  ½ ounce cashews, unsalted (1 meat/beans plus 1 oil)
  1 Incredibly Good Chocolate Chip and Walnut Cookie* (80 extra calories)

Day 2

Breakfast

  1 toasted whole-wheat English muffin (2 grains)
  2 teaspoons trans fat–free margarine (2 oils)
  1 clementine (½ cup fruit)
  1 cup skim milk (1 milk/yogurt/cheese)

Lunch

2 slices whole-wheat bread (2 grains)

2 slices fresh roasted turkey breast (2 meat/beans)

1 slice Swiss cheese (½ milk/yogurt/cheese)

2 leaves romaine lettuce (¼ cup vegetables)

2 slices tomato (¼ cup vegetables)

1 teaspoon mayonnaise (1 oil)

1 teaspoon Dijon mustard (0 extra calories)

Dinner

Chipotle Lime Seared Salmon Fajitas* (½ cup vegetables, 1½ grains, 4 meat/beans plus 1½ oils)

Sweet and Tangy Asparagus* (about 6 spears: 1 cup vegetables plus 1 oil)

Snacks/Desserts

½ cup (4 ounces) low-fat plain yogurt (½ milk/yogurt/cheese plus 30 extra calories) mixed with 1 cup sliced strawberries (1 cup fruit)

2 chewy chocolate chip cookies (120 extra calories)

1 cup skim milk (1 milk/yogurt/cheese)

Day 3

Breakfast

Southwestern Egg White Breakfast Burrito* (1 grain, ½ meat/beans, ¼ milk/yogurt/cheese plus ½ cup vegetables)

1 cup raspberries (1 cup fruit)

1 cup skim milk (1 milk/yogurt/cheese)

Lunch

Sandwich:

1 2-ounce whole-wheat sub roll (2 grains)

2 ounces light tuna, canned (2 meat/beans)

2 teaspoons mayonnaise (2 oils)

1 cup baby carrots (1 cup vegetables) dipped in 1 tablespoon creamy Italian salad dressing (1 oil)

1 green apple (1 cup fruit)

Dinner

Oven-fried chicken drumsticks* (2 grains 4½ meat/beans plus
1 milk/yogurt/cheese)

1 sweet potato (1 cup vegetables)

2 teaspoons trans fat–free margarine (2 oils)

Snacks/Desserts

2 ounces natural Swiss cheese, cut into slivers (1 milk/yogurt/cheese
plus 90 extra calories) and 10 small whole-wheat low-fat crackers
(1 grain)

½ cup all-natural light ice cream (110 extra calories)

Day 4

Breakfast

Super strawberry smoothie* (1 cup fruit, ½ milk/yogurt/cheese,
1 grain plus 60 extra calories)

1 slice whole-wheat toast (1 grain)

1 teaspoon trans fat–free margarine (1 oil)

Lunch

Sandwich:

   3 ounces grilled chicken breast (3 meat/beans)

   1 ounce mozzarella cheese, low moisture, part skim (½
   milk/yogurt/cheese)

   ¼ avocado, sliced (¼ cup fruit plus 2 oils)

   2 slices (2 ounces) Italian bread (2 grains)

½ cup cantaloupe cubes (½ cup fruit)

Dinner

Whole-Wheat Penne with Meatless Bolognese* (1 oil, 2 grains
plus 1 cup vegetables)

2 tablespoons grated parmesan cheese (½ milk/yogurt/cheese)

Snacks/Desserts

½ cup (snack-size) sugar-free chocolate pudding (½
milk/yogurt/cheese)

1 ounce unsalted raw cashews (2 meat/beans plus 2 oils)

1 cup baby carrots (1 cup vegetables)

1 cup skim milk (1 milk/yogurt/cheese)

Day 5

Breakfast

½ cup cooked oatmeal (1 grain) plus 1 teaspoon trans fat–free
margarine (1 oil)

1 cup sliced strawberries (1 cup fruit)

1 hard-boiled egg (1 meat/beans)

1 cup skim milk (1 milk/yogurt/cheese)

Lunch

Cold Peanut, Noodle, and Vegetable Salad* (1 cup vegetables,
2 grains plus 1 meat/beans)

Dinner

Tempting Turkey Meatloaf* (½ cup vegetables, ¼ grain plus 4
meat/beans)

1 cup cooked peas and carrots (1 cup vegetables) and 1 teaspoon
trans fat–free margarine (1 oil)

½ cup wild rice (1 grain) made with 1 teaspoon canola oil (1 oil)

1 cup skim milk (1 milk/yogurt/cheese)

Snacks/Desserts

1 small peach (½ cup fruit)

2 ounces reduced-fat cheddar cheese wedge (1 milk/yogurt/cheese)

3 cups popcorn (1 grain) made with 2 teaspoons canola oil (2 oil)

Day 6

Breakfast

1 toasted whole-wheat English muffin (2 grains) topped with ½
cup low-fat ricotta cheese (1 milk/yogurt/cheese) and ¼ cup
raisins (½ cup fruit)

½ cup (4 ounces) orange juice (½ cup fruit)

Lunch

Tuna melt:

> 2 ounces canned light tuna (2 meat/beans) and 1 teaspoon
> mayonnaise (1 oil)
>
> 1 slice American cheese (½ milk/yogurt/cheese)
>
> 1 small whole-wheat pita, toasted (1 grain)
>
> 2 romaine lettuce leaves (¼ cup vegetables)
>
> 2 slices tomato (¼ cup vegetables)

1 green apple (1 cup fruit)

1 cup skim milk (1 milk/yogurt/cheese)

Dinner

3 ounces sirloin steak (3 meat/beans), pan fried with 2 teaspoons
vegetable oil (2 oils)

Couscous with Asparagus, Orange, and Mint* (⅓ cup vegetables,
2 grains plus ½ oil)

Snacks/Desserts

1 cup raw carrots and pepper slices (1 cup vegetables) and 2
tablespoons ranch salad dressing, reduced fat (2 oils)

Day 7

Breakfast

2 small banana pancakes (mix ⅓ cup complete pancake mix and
⅓ cup water with 1 ripe banana, mashed) (2 grains plus 1 cup
fruit)

1 tablespoon light syrup (25 extra calories)

2 teaspoons trans fat–free margarine (2 oils)

1 cup skim milk (1 milk/yogurt/cheese)

Lunch

Zesty Three-Bean Salad* (¼ cup vegetables, 2 meat/beans plus 1
oil)

1 toasted whole-wheat pita (1 grain)

Dinner

Penne with Shrimp and Broccoli Rabe* (1¼ cup vegetables, 2 grains, 2 meat/beans plus 1½ oils)

Snacks/Desserts

Cheesy nachos:

1 ounce baked tortilla chips (1 grain or 120 extra calories) topped with 2 ounces melted low-fat cheddar cheese (1 milk/yogurt/cheese) dipped in ¼ cup salsa (½ cup vegetables)

1 cup chocolate vanilla swirl pudding (1 milk/yogurt/cheese plus 60 extra calories)

1 cup blueberries (1 cup fruit)

Day 8

Breakfast

Egg in a cup:

1 egg, scrambled (1 meat/beans) with 1 teaspoon trans fat–free margarine (1 oil)

1 slice whole-wheat toast (1 grain)

1 teaspoon trans fat–free margarine (1 oil)

1 cup skim milk (1 milk/yogurt/cheese)

½ cup (4 ounces) orange juice (½ cup fruit)

Lunch

Turkey salad:

2 cups romaine lettuce (1 cup vegetables)

2 ounces fresh roasted turkey breast (2 meat/beans)

¼ cup (1 ounce) walnut halves (1 meat/beans plus 1 oil)

1 pear, chopped (1 cup fruit)

2 tablespoons Italian dressing (2 oils)

¼ cup croutons (½ grain)

1 whole-wheat pita, toasted (1½ grains)

1 teaspoon trans fat–free margarine (1 oil)

Dinner

One-Pot Vegetable Beef Chili* (3 meat/beans plus 2 cups vegetables)
½ cup brown rice (1 grain)

Snacks/Desserts

1 ounce pretzels (1 grain)
½ ounce dark chocolate (75 extra calories)

Day 9

Breakfast

Parfait:

1 cup low-fat plain yogurt (1 milk/yogurt/cheese plus 60 extra calories)
1 cup sliced strawberries (1 cup fruit)
2 tablespoons walnut halves (1 meat/beans plus 1 oil)
¼ cup low-fat granola (1 grain)

Lunch

Tuna salad wrap:

3 ounces canned light tuna (3 meat/beans) mixed in a bowl with ½ cup shredded carrots (½ cup vegetables), ½ cup shredded cabbage (½ cup vegetables), 2 teaspoons mayonnaise (2 oils) plus 1 teaspoon Dijon mustard (0 extra calories)
1 7- to 8-inch whole-wheat flour tortilla (2 grains)
½ cup red grapes (½ cup fruit)
1 cup skim milk (1 milk/yogurt/cheese)

Dinner

Chessy Chickpea Pesto Pasta* (2 grains, 1 meat/beans, ¼ milk/yogurt/cheese plus 1 oil)

Snacks/Desserts

3 graham cracker squares (1 grain)
1 cup skim milk (1 milk/yogurt/cheese)
1 cup cucumber slices (1 cup vegetables) dipped in 1 tablespoon Italian salad dressing (1 oil)

Day 10

Breakfast
1 cup cooked oatmeal (2 grains) topped with ½ cup fresh blueberries (½ cup fruit)

1 cup skim milk (1 milk/yogurt/cheese)

Lunch
2 cups mixed salad greens (1 cup vegetables)

3 ounces grilled chicken breast (3 meat/beans)

½ cup cherry tomatoes (½ cup vegetables)

2 tablespoons balsamic vinaigrette salad dressing (2 oils)

1 small apple (1 cup fruit)

Dinner
1 cup (2 ounces) cooked spaghetti (2 grains) topped with 1 cup cooked broccoli florets (1 cup vegetables) and 2 ounces melted part-skim mozzarella cheese (1 milk/yogurt/cheese plus 90 extra calories)

Snacks/Desserts
Banana Nut Loaf Cake* (1 grain, 1 cup fruit plus 80 extra calories)

1 cup skim milk (1 milk/yogurt/cheese)

½ peanut butter and jelly sandwich:

    2 tablespoons natural peanut butter (2 meat/beans plus 2 oils)

    1 tablespoon sugar-free jelly (5 extra calories)

    1 slice whole-wheat bread (1 grain)

Day 11

Breakfast
1 cup oat bran flakes cereal (2 grains)

1 sliced banana (1 cup fruit)

1 cup skim milk (1 milk/yogurt/cheese)

Lunch
Curried Split Pea Soup* (1 cup vegetables plus 4 meat/beans)

1 toasted whole-wheat pita (1½ grains)

1 teaspoon trans fat–free margarine (1 oil)

Dinner

1 slice 14-inch pizza, thick crust (2 grains, ¼ cup vegetables, 1 milk/yogurt/cheese plus 1 oil)

2 cups mixed green salad with ¼ cup cut-up tomatoes and ¼ cup pepper strips (1½ cup vegetables) topped with 2 tablespoons Italian salad dressing (2 oils)

Snacks/Desserts

1 cup low-fat yogurt (1 milk/yogurt/cheese plus 60 extra calories)

1 cup pineapple chunks (1 cup fruit)

½ ounce nuts (1 meat/beans plus 1 oils)

Day 12

Breakfast

1 slice whole-wheat toast (1 grain)

1 teaspoon trans fat–free margarine (1 oil)

Vegetable scrambled eggs made in a pan with:

    1 large egg (1 meat/beans)

    1 large egg white (¼ meat/beans)

    ½ cup chopped bell pepper (½ cup vegetables)

    ½ cup low-fat shredded cheddar cheese (1 milk/yogurt/cheese)

    2 teaspoons canola oil (2 oils)

1 cup skim milk (1 milk/yogurt/cheese)

Lunch

Turkey burger:

    3-ounce turkey burger (made with lean ground turkey) (3 meat/beans)

    1 kaiser roll (2 grains)

    2 romaine lettuce leaves (¼ cup vegetables)

    2 slices tomato (¼ cup vegetables)

    1 teaspoon catsup (5 extra calories)

1 cup fresh fruit salad (1 cup fruit)

Dinner

1 lean pork chop, broiled (3 meat/beans)

1 cup lightly sauteed mixed vegetables made with:

½ cup summer squash (½ cup vegetables)

½ cup chopped tomatoes (½ cup vegetables)

¼ cup chopped white onion (¼ cup vegetables)

2 teaspoons olive oil (2 oils)

¼ teaspoon garlic powder (0 extra calories)

1 cup wild rice (2 grains) topped with 1 teaspoon trans fat–free margarine (1 oil)

Snacks/Desserts

1 green apple, sliced (1 cup fruit)

1 cup skim milk (1 milk/yogurt/cheese)

3 gingersnap cookies (90 extra calories)

Day 13

Breakfast

1 toasted whole-wheat English muffin (2 grains)

2 teaspoons trans fat–free margarine (2 oils)

8 ounces low-fat vanilla yogurt (1 milk/yogurt/cheese plus 60 extra calories)

Lunch

Soft Tofu Tacos* (1 grain, ½ cup vegetables, 1 meat/beans, ¼ milk/yogurt/cheese plus 40 extra calories)

2 clementines (1 cup fruit)

Dinner

3 ounces broiled flank steak (3 meat/beans)

½ medium (about 3 ounces) baked potato (½ cup vegetables) topped with 1 tablespoon reduced-fat sour cream (25 extra calories), ¼ cup (or 1 ounce) low-fat shredded cheddar cheese (½ milk/yogurt/cheese) plus 1 teaspoon trans fat–free margarine (1 oil)

1 cup steamed broccoli spears (1 cup vegetables)

Snacks/Desserts

1 cup skim milk (1 milk/yogurt/cheese)

¼ cup raisins (½ cup fruit) mixed with 1 ounce raw cashews, unsalted (2 meat/beans plus 2 oils), and ¼ cup low-fat granola (1 grain)

5 reduced-fat whole-grain crackers (1 grain)

Day 14

Breakfast

1 cup Multigrain Cheerios (1 grain)

½ cup fresh sliced strawberries (½ cup fruit)

½ cup (4 ounces) skim milk (½ milk/yogurt/cheese)

1 hard-boiled large egg (1 meat/beans)

Lunch

Bean and cheese burrito:

   ½ cup cooked lentils (2 meat/beans)

   1 large whole-wheat flour tortilla (2 grains)

   ¼ cup (1 ounce) low-fat shredded cheddar cheese (½ milk/yogurt/cheese)

   ½ cup salsa (1 cup vegetables)

1 medium pear, sliced (1 cup fruit)

Dinner

Spinach and Sausage Lasagna* (2 grains, 1½ meat/beans, 1 milk/yogurt/cheese plus ¼ cup vegetables)

1½ cups sliced peppers, carrots and celery (1½ cup vegetables) plus 2 tablespoons Italian salad dressing (2 oils)

Snacks/Desserts

1 Tropical Oatmeal Raisin Cookies* (80 extra calories)

1 cup skim milk (1 milk/yogurt/cheese)

3 cups popcorn (1 grain) made with 2 teaspoons canola oil (2 oils)

1 ounce mixed nuts, dry roasted, unsalted (2 meat/beans plus 2 oils)

15

Family-Friendly Recipes

Breakfasts

Southwestern Egg White Breakfast Burritos

These burritos make a satisfying and tasty breakfast that the whole family will love. They're low in fat but high in flavor—a great way to incorporate vegetables and whole grains into your day.

6 egg whites
2 tablespoons skim milk
nonstick cooking spray
½ cup diced red bell pepper
¼ cup chopped scallions
½ teaspoon southwestern seasoning blend, such as Emeril's
¼ teaspoon salt
¼ teaspoon pepper
¼ cup low-fat shredded cheddar cheese
4 8-inch whole-wheat tortillas
1 cup salsa

Total preparation and cooking time: 20 minutes

Makes 4 servings.

Nutrition information per serving:
Calories: 140
Fat: 1.5 g
Saturated fat: 0 g
Cholesterol: 0 mg
Sodium: 700 mg
Carbohydrate: 27 g
Fiber: 2 g
Sugar: 4 g
Protein: 11 g

In a bowl combine the egg whites and skim milk. Spray a nonstick medium sauté pan with the

Southwestern Egg White Breakfast Burritos *(continued)*

nonstick cooking spray. Add the bell pepper and
scallions and sauté over medium heat for 5 to 6
minutes until softened. Add the egg mixture,
southwestern seasoning blend, salt, and pepper.
Cook until the egg mixture is firm and fluffy. Add
the cheese and stir occasionally for 1 to 2 minutes
until the cheese is melted. Place the tortillas in the
microwave for 10 to 15 seconds until lightly
warmed. Divide the egg mixture evenly onto the
tortillas, fold the edges in, and roll them up. Serve
with salsa.

Cook's Tip: For variety, you can replace the
red bell pepper and scallions with tomatoes and
onions.

Silver Dollar Sweet Potato Pancakes

This recipe is one of my family's favorites. Sweet potatoes add flavor and texture to your usual pancakes. They also provide tons of vitamin A as well as fiber and help you meet your daily quota for vegetables. These pancakes are easy to prepare and provide a wonderful opportunity to get your kids in the kitchen.

1 medium sweet potato
nonstick cooking spray
⅔ cup pancake and waffle mix, complete, dry
⅛ teaspoon ground cinnamon
¾ cup water
2 teaspoons powdered sugar

Total preparation and cooking time: 15 to 20 minutes

Makes 2 servings (3 pancakes per serving).

Nutrition information per serving:
Calories: 230
Fat: 2.5 g
Saturated fat: 0.5 g
Cholesterol: 10 mg
Sodium: 500 mg
Carbohydrate: 47 g
Fiber: 3 g
Sugar: 14 g
Protein: 6 g

Clean the sweet potato, poke it with a fork, wrap it in a paper towel, and microwave it for 7 or 8 minutes or until you can easily put a fork in it. Set it aside. Spray a griddle or a large pan with the cooking spray, and set it on medium heat. Pour the pancake and waffle mix into a large bowl, along with the cinnamon, and add the water to the mix (add more water for fluffier pancakes, less for denser pancakes). Scoop out the sweet potato and add it to the mix. Combine the ingredients until the desired texture is achieved. Cook the pancakes on the griddle or in the large pan (you can make about six silver dollar pancakes). Watch the pancakes carefully and flip them after 3 or 4 minutes or when they're firm. Cook them another 3 or 4 minutes, and remove them from the heat promptly. Stack them, sprinkle with powdered sugar, and serve.

Cook's Tip: You can use another sweet potato and make some pancakes to freeze and pop in the microwave oven for a quick and easy breakfast later in the week. These pancakes can also make a hearty side dish for dinner.

Papa's Grilled Cheese French Toast

When my dad, otherwise known as Papa, comes for a weekend visit, he makes this recipe for his grandsons, Spencer and Eli, who devour it. Not only does this dish taste delicious, but it's a fine way to incorporate some high-quality protein from eggs, not to mention fiber and whole grains from the whole-wheat bread.

nonstick cooking spray
2 eggs (1 yolk removed)
2 teaspoons trans fat–free margarine or vegetable oil spread
4 slices whole-wheat bread
2 slices American cheese

Total preparation and cooking time: 20 minutes

Makes 2 servings.

Nutrition information per serving:
Calories: 290
Fat: 14 g
Saturated fat: 5 g
Cholesterol: 125 mg
Sodium: 740 mg
Carbohydrate: 28 g
Fiber: 4 g
Sugar: 4 g
Protein: 15 g

Spray a griddle with the nonstick cooking spray. Set on medium heat. Crack the eggs into a medium bowl, remove one yolk, and beat. Spread the margarine on one side of each slice of bread. Then dip the bread, one slice at a time, until completely coated with egg. When the griddle is hot, place the bread on it. After about 2 minutes, add 1 slice of cheese to two of the slices of bread on the griddle. Take the two pieces of bread without the cheese and flip them onto each slice of cheese to make two sandwiches. Cook for 2 more minutes and flip until both sides of each sandwich are light brown. Cut into fours and serve.

Cook's Tip: For even more flavor, you can use cheddar cheese instead of American cheese. This dish tastes great with a cup of skim milk. It can also be served for lunch with a side of fruit salad.

Salads and Soups

Cold Peanut, Noodle, and Vegetable Salad

This salad has a lot of crunch and provides a hearty and flavorful meal packed with protein and healthful monounsaturated fats.

8 ounces whole-wheat linguine noodles
1 teaspoon fresh grated ginger
1 clove minced garlic
¼ cup natural chunky peanut butter
2 tablespoons rice wine vinegar
2 tablespoons low-sodium soy sauce
½ teaspoon crushed red pepper flakes (optional)
½ cup chopped fresh scallions
½ cup chopped fresh cilantro
1 cup cucumber, cut in strips
½ cup shredded carrots
2 cups shredded romaine lettuce

Total preparation and cooking time: 30 minutes

Makes 4 servings.

Nutrition information per serving:
Calories: 330
Fat: 9 g
Saturated fat: 1 g
Cholesterol: 0 mg
Sodium: 350 mg
Carbohydrate: 52 g
Fiber: 10 g
Sugar: 5 g
Protein: 13 g

Cook the noodles according to the package directions. Drain and rinse with cold water to stop cooking and then cool. While the noodles are cooking, in a large bowl whisk together the ginger, garlic, peanut butter, rice wine vinegar, soy sauce and crushed red pepper (if desired) until well blended. Toss in the noodles and then add the scallions, cilantro, cucumber, carrots, and lettuce. Toss together until all the noodles and vegetables are coated. Garnish with additional chopped scallions and the shredded carrots if desired.
Serve cold.

Cook's Tip: You can substitute penne to provide added texture.

Zesty Three-Bean Salad

This delicious side dish provides a perfect vehicle for protein, fiber, and vegetables. It's a simple dish that takes little time to prepare.

2 tablespoons extra-virgin olive oil
2 tablespoons lime juice
2 tablespoons light teriyaki sauce
2 teaspoons lime zest
2 tablespoons chopped cilantro
1 15-ounce can chickpeas
1 15-ounce can black beans
1 15-ounce can kidney beans
½ cup finely diced red onion
1 cup diced carrots
1 cup cherry tomatoes, cut in half
salt and pepper

Total preparation and cooking time: 15 minutes

Makes 9 1-cup servings.

Nutrition information per serving:
Calories: 170
Fat: 4.5 g
Saturated fat: 0 g
Cholesterol: 0 mg
Sodium: 470 mg
Carbohydrate: 24 g
Fiber: 7 g
Sugar: 4 g
Protein: 8 g

In a large bowl combine the olive oil with the lime juice, teriyaki sauce, lime zest, and cilantro. Toss in the chickpeas, black beans, kidney beans, red onion, carrots, and cherry tomatoes. Add salt and pepper to taste. Serve.

Cook's Tip: This dish gets even better if made ahead and chilled for 30 minutes or longer before serving. It can also be consumed in a larger portion as a main meal.

Curried Split Pea Soup

This soup, loaded with fiber and protein, provides an easy way to eat your vegetables. It's extremely filling and has just the right amount of kick to please your palate.

nonstick cooking spray
1 diced green pepper
1 cup finely diced onion
4 cloves minced garlic
1 cup diced celery
1¼ cups diced carrots
1¼ cups diced parsnips
½ teaspoon kosher salt
2 teaspoons curry powder
1 teaspoon ground ginger
¾ pound dried split peas
4 cups vegetable stock
4 cups water
¼ cup chopped parsley

Total preparation and cooking time: 3½ hours

Makes 6 servings.

Nutrition information per serving:

Calories: 260
Fat: 1.5 g
Saturated fat: 0 g
Cholesterol: 0 mg
Sodium: 430 mg
Carbohydrate: 48 g
Fiber: 18 g
Sugar: 9 g
Protein: 16 g

Spray a large pot, over medium heat, with the nonstick cooking spray. Sauté the green peppers, onions, minced garlic, celery, carrots, and parsnips for 5 minutes until slightly softened. Add the salt, curry powder, and ginger, and cook an additional 3 minutes until well combined. Add the split peas, vegetable stock, and water. Bring to a boil and stir occasionally for 5 minutes, reduce heat, and simmer for 3 hours, stirring occasionally. Add the parsley and season with additional salt and pepper if desired.

Cook's Tip: Serve with toasted mini pita pockets.

Fruity Chicken Salad

This refreshing chicken salad, created by Paolo Casagranda, the chef at Mezzaluna, one of my favorite local Italian restaurants, is a great-tasting year-round dish.

2 small red apples, cut into strips
1½ cups canned corn kernels
½ cup golden raisins
½ cup diced celery
½ cup diced fennel
1 pint red cherry tomatoes, cut into quarters
1½ avocados, diced into ½-inch cubes
7 cups of greens such as arugula, frisée, or radicchio, lightly chopped
5 medium organic chicken or turkey breasts, lightly pounded
2 tablespoons balsamic vinegar
6 tablespoons extra-virgin olive oil
1 teaspoon sea salt
freshly ground pepper(optional)
juice of 2 lemons
½ teaspoon Dijon mustard

Total preparation and cooking time: 35 minutes

Makes 10 servings.

Nutrition information per serving:
Calories: 260
Fat: 14 g
Saturated fat: 2 g
Cholesterol: 35 mg
Sodium: 300 mg
Carbohydrate: 20 g
Fiber: 5 g
Sugar: 10 g
Protein: 16 g

Mix together the apples, corn, raisins, celery, fennel, tomatoes, avocados, and the greens in a large mixing bowl. Marinate the chicken breast in the balsamic vinegar, 1½ tablespoons of the extra-virgin oil, and salt and pepper for approximately 5 minutes. Brush a large pan with extra-virgin olive oil and set on medium to high heat. Grill the breasts on each side for 3 to 4 minutes and set aside. Once the chicken is cool to the touch, chop into ½-inch cubes. Add the chicken to the prepared salad ingredients. In a separate bowl, mix together the lemon juice, Dijon mustard, remaining extra-virgin olive oil, and salt and pepper. Add the dressing to the salad. Toss gently.

Cook's Tip: In the summer, you can add fresh corn kernels for more pleasurable sweetness and crunch.

Tangy Apple Salad

This recipe, created by my friend Linda Quinn, M.S., R.D., for the New York Apple Association, is a refreshing and easy way to make a midday snack packed with protein and fiber to fill you up and give you energy.

¾ cup (6 ounces) plain, low-fat yogurt
1 tablespoon orange marmalade
freshly ground black pepper to taste
1 head romaine lettuce (makes about 6 cups shredded lettuce)
3 apples of your choice
¼ cup sliced almonds

Total preparation and cooking time: 10 minutes

Makes 5 servings.

Nutrition information per serving:
Calories: 145
Fat: 4.5 g
Saturated fat: 0.5 g
Cholesterol: 0 mg
Sodium: 55 mg
Carbohydrate: 26 g
Fiber: 4 g
Sugar: 20 g
Protein: 4 g

In a small bowl, mix the yogurt with the marmalade and pepper to make the dressing. Tear the lettuce into bite-size pieces and set aside. Cut the apples into small cubes. In a large bowl, mix the lettuce, apples, almonds, and dressing. Serve immediately.

BB's Garlic Chicken Salad

This salad is very flavorful because of the marinade—my mom's creation—used to make the chicken. It's packed with protein and fiber, fills you up, and keeps you energized midday.

1 pound chicken breast, skinless and boneless
lemon juice (from 1½ fresh lemons)
1 lemon rind, grated
3 cloves fresh chopped garlic
1 tablespoon fresh chopped parsley
1 tablespoon fresh chopped cilantro
2 tablespoons olive oil
nonstick cooking spray
4 cups romaine lettuce
1 cup shredded carrots
8 tablespoons low-fat salad dressing

Total preparation and cooking time: 1 hour and 20 minutes (including 1 hour of marinating)

Makes 4 servings.

Nutrition information per serving:
Calories: 250
Fat: 11 g
Saturated fat: 1.5 g
Cholesterol: 65 mg
Sodium: 320 mg
Carbohydrate: 8 g
Fiber: 2 g
Sugar: 3 g
Protein: 27 g

Cut the chicken into 4 pieces. In a large bowl, combine the lemon juice, lemon rind, garlic, parsley, cilantro, and olive oil to make a paste. Place the chicken in the bowl with the marinade and mix together. Cover the chicken and refrigerate for 1 hour. Then grill the chicken for 5 minutes or so on each side, or sauté the chicken in a nonstick skillet for 3 to 4 minutes on each side or until thoroughly cooked. Wash the romaine thoroughly and tear into bite-size pieces. When the chicken is thoroughly cooked, cut it into slices and mix with the romaine. Blend in the carrots and salad dressing and serve.

Cook's Tip: This chicken can be served alone, hot alongside broccoli, brussels sprouts or green beans, or on toasted Italian bread.

Main Courses

Extra Creamy Macaroni and Cheese

Kids love mac and cheese, and secretly, so do adults. This one is almost guilt free and tastes great.

8 ounces elbow macaroni, preferably whole wheat
1¼ cups skim milk
1 tablespoon flour
2 cups (8 ounces) low-fat cheddar cheese, shredded
⅓ cup grated parmesan cheese
2 teaspoons Tabasco sauce
2 teaspoons Dijon mustard
1 teaspoon paprika
¼ teaspoon salt
¼ teaspoon pepper
nonstick cooking spray

Total preparation and cooking time: 30 minutes

Makes 4 servings.

Nutrition information per serving:
Calories: 360
Fat: 7 g
Saturated fat: 4 g
Cholesterol: 20 mg
Sodium: 680 mg
Carbohydrate: 49 g
Fiber: 5 g
Sugar: 4 g
Protein: 28 g

Cook the macaroni according to the package directions, drain, and set aside in a bowl. In the same pot, over medium heat, bring the milk to a simmer. Reduce the heat to low and whisk in the flour until slightly thickened. Whisk in 1¾ cups of the cheddar and the parmesan cheese, Tabasco sauce, Dijon mustard, paprika, salt, and pepper. Cook about 3 to 4 minutes until smooth and creamy. Stir in the macaroni. Spray a 1½-quart baking dish with the nonstick cooking spray and transfer the macaroni to the dish. Sprinkle with the remaining ¼ cup cheddar cheese, and broil for 1 to 2 minutes until the cheese is melted and lightly golden.

Cook's Tip: You can add broccoli florets for added crunch, not to mention extra calcium.

Cheesy Chickpea Pesto Pasta

If you love pesto but don't like all the fat and sodium that is typically found in the jarred versions, try this quick and easy variation. It's loaded with protein without as much fat and sodium.

Pesto Sauce:
- 3 cups basil leaves, washed and dried
- 1 15½-ounce can (about 2 cups) chickpeas, drained and rinsed
- 2 cloves garlic
- ½ teaspoon kosher salt
- ¼ teaspoon pepper
- ½ cup grated parmesan cheese
- ¼ cup extra-virgin olive oil
- ¼ cup water
- 1 pound fusilli or rotini pasta
- 2 tablespoons extra-virgin olive oil
- additional grated cheese (optional)

Total preparation and cooking time: 30 minutes.

Makes 8 servings.

Nutrition information per serving:
Calories: 370
Fat: 14 g
Saturated fat: 2.5 g
Cholesterol: 5 mg
Sodium: 280 mg
Carbohydrate: 51 g
Fiber: 5 g
Sugar: 4 g
Protein: 13 g

Place all the pesto sauce ingredients in a food processor. Purée for approximately 2 minutes until the mixture forms a thick paste. Store, refrigerated, in an airtight container until ready to use.

Boil the pasta according to the package directions. Drain and reserve ¼ cup of the pasta water. Toss the pasta with the extra-virgin olive oil, pesto sauce, and pasta water until well blended. Garnish with the additional grated cheese if desired.

Cook's Tip: This pesto sauce is a tasty topping over whole-wheat pasta or the base for a delicious dip.

Crunchy Chicken Nuggets

This dish, straight from the pages of my last book, So What Can I Eat?! *(Wiley, 2006), is one of my family's favorites. Over the years I have played with the ingredients, and the following combination is always a winner in my home.*

nonstick cooking spray
1 pound chicken breast, skinless and boneless
2 cups cornflakes cereal
½ cup breadcrumbs
¼ cup grated parmesan cheese
½ teaspoon garlic powder
½ teaspoon onion powder
4 egg whites
1 tablespoon olive oil

Total preparation and cooking time: 30 minutes

Makes 4 servings.

Nutrition information per serving:
Calories: 300
Fat: 7 g
Saturated fat: 2 g
Cholesterol: 70 mg
Sodium: 410 mg
Carbohydrate: 23 g
Fiber: 1 g
Sugar: 3 g
Protein: 35 g

Preheat oven to 350 degrees F. Use the nonstick cooking spray to coat a nonstick baking sheet and set aside. Divide the chicken breast into 8 equal pieces. Pour the cornflakes, breadcrumbs, parmesan cheese, garlic powder, and onion powder into a large plastic bag. Seal the bag, removing most of the air, and mash with your fist until the contents are finely ground. Pour the mixture onto a large plate. Beat the egg whites and olive oil in a medium bowl. Dip the chicken into the egg and olive oil mixture and then into the cornflake mixture, coating each piece entirely. Place the coated chicken onto the baking sheet. Bake for 8 to 10 minutes. Serve.

Cook's Tip: This chicken goes well with roasted red potatoes and a green vegetable. It can also be served cold and sliced to top salad greens. To make this into a flavorful appetizer, cut the chicken into bite-size pieces and add ½ cup finely chopped raw cashews to the cornflake and breadcrumb mixture.

Tempting Turkey Meatloaf

This meatloaf is the ultimate comfort food, sure to satisfy even picky eaters.

nonstick cooking spray
2¼ pounds ground white meat turkey
1 egg, lightly beaten
¼ cup water
1 cup onion, finely chopped
2 cloves minced garlic
2 teaspoons fresh thyme
1 tablespoon fresh chopped parsley
¼ cup diced carrots
¼ cup diced celery
½ cup plain breadcrumbs
2 tablespoons Worcestershire sauce
½ cup low-fat shredded cheddar cheese
½ teaspoon salt
¼ teaspoon pepper
2 tablespoons ketchup

Total preparation and cooking time: 1 hour and 15 minutes

Makes 8 servings.

Nutrition information per serving:
Calories: 240
Fat: 10 g
Saturated fat: 3 g
Cholesterol: 100 mg
Sodium: 430 mg
Carbohydrate: 10 g
Fiber: 1 g
Sugar: 3 g
Protein: 29 g

Preheat oven to 375 degrees F. Coat a 9 by 5-inch loaf pan with the nonstick cooking spray. Combine the turkey with the egg and water until well moistened. Add the onion, garlic, thyme, parsley, carrots, celery, breadcrumbs, Worcestershire sauce, cheddar cheese, salt, and pepper, and mix together until all ingredients are well combined. Gently press the turkey mixture into the loaf pan. Bake for 30 minutes, brushing with the ketchup twice. Continue baking until fully cooked and a thermometer reads 165 degrees F, about 30 more minutes. Let the loaf rest for 5 minutes. Transfer it to a platter and serve.

Cook's Tip: This meatloaf tastes great cold the next day on a sandwich with sliced tomato.

Soft Tofu Tacos

These vegetarian tacos are quite tasty and a satisfying way to incorporate high-quality protein without a lot of saturated fat or cholesterol.

nonstick cooking spray
8 ounces extra-firm tofu, diced into ½-inch pieces, (about 1 cup)
2 tablespoons low-sodium taco seasoning mix
½ cup diced red pepper
¼ cup diced red onion
2 tablespoons chopped fresh cilantro
½ cup water
4 8-inch whole-wheat tortillas
½ cup shredded low-fat cheddar cheese
¼ cup reduced-fat sour cream
1 cup shredded romaine lettuce
¼ cup (4 tablespoons) salsa

Total preparation and cooking time: 30 minutes

Makes 4 servings (4 tacos).

Nutrition information per serving:
Calories: 210
Fat: 7 g
Saturated fat: 2.5 g
Cholesterol: 10 mg
Sodium: 550 mg
Carbohydrate: 28 g
Fiber: 3 g
Sugar: 3 g
Protein: 14 g

Lightly coat a 10-inch nonstick skillet with the nonstick cooking spray and heat on medium setting. Add the tofu and taco seasoning mix and cook for 2 to 3 minutes until slightly brown. Add the red pepper, red onion, and cilantro, and cook for an additional 2 to 3 minutes. Add the water and allow it to be absorbed (about 3 minutes). Turn off the heat. Warm the tortillas in the microwave on high for 1 minute. Place approximately 3 tablespoons of the tofu mixture in the center of each tortilla. Top each one with 2 tablespoons of cheddar cheese and 1 tablespoon of sour cream. Divide the lettuce evenly on each taco and top with 1 tablespoon of salsa.

Cook's Tip: Brown rice or black beans round out this meal nicely.

Oven-Fried Chicken Drumsticks

These tasty oven-fried drumsticks are crisp and flavorful, likely to appeal to kids (and parents) of all ages.

nonstick cooking spray
⅔ cup buttermilk
1 tablespoon chopped parsley
1 teaspoon cajun seasoning
1 teaspoon dried thyme
¼ teaspoon salt
8 skinless chicken drumsticks
3 egg whites
2 tablespoons water
½ cup crushed cornflakes
¼ cup whole-wheat flour

Total preparation and cooking time: 1 hour and 10 minutes

Makes 4 servings (2 drumsticks per serving).

Nutrition information per serving:
Calories: 220
Fat: 5 g
Saturated fat: 1.5 g
Cholesterol: 95 mg
Sodium: 500 mg
Carbohydrate: 11 g
Fiber: 1 g
Sugar: 3 g
Protein: 31 g

Prepare a roasting pan with aluminum foil and spray a wire rack with the nonstick cooking spray. Preheat the oven to 400 degrees F. In a large bowl, mix together the buttermilk, parsley, cajun seasoning, thyme, and salt. Add the chicken and soak for 10 minutes. Beat the egg whites in a bowl with the water. Set aside. In a separate bowl, combine the cornflakes and whole-wheat flour and set aside. Remove the chicken drumsticks from the buttermilk and dip into the egg white mixture. Roll the drumsticks in the cornflake mixture until coated. Place on the wire rack, and repeat until all the chicken is done. Cook the chicken for 40 to 45 minutes until golden, the thermometer reads 170 degrees F, and the meat is no longer pink near the bone. If necessary, cover the chicken with foil to prevent burning.

Cook's Tip: You can serve this with wild rice and a green or orange vegetable.

Spaghetti with Eggplant, Mozzarella, and Tomato

This is my favorite dish at Mezzaluna, a local Italian restaurant. Chef Paolo Casagranda makes this simple dish and it always tastes so fresh and delicious, especially in the spring when eggplant and tomatoes are in season.

2 medium eggplants, cut into small cubes
½ teaspoon sea salt
½ cup extra-virgin olive oil
2 large chopped garlic cloves
1 16-ounce can peeled Italian tomatoes, drained
1½ pounds plum tomatoes, chopped
4 large basil leaves, sliced in half
½ teaspoon coarse salt
freshly ground pepper (optional)
1 pound dry spaghetti, preferably Italian imported
2 cups fresh mozzarella cheese, cut into small cubes

Total preparation and cooking time: 1 hour

Makes 8 servings.

Nutrition information per serving:
Calories: 440
Fat: 17 g
Saturated fat: 6 g
Cholesterol: 20 mg
Sodium: 630 mg
Carbohydrate: 57 g
Fiber: 8 g
Sugar: 8 g
Protein: 16 g

Place the prepared eggplant in a strainer. Sprinkle it with the sea salt. Toss gently and set aside for approximately 20 minutes to fully drain its water content. Remove the eggplant from the strainer. Pat dry. Heat a large pan over medium heat. Add the extra-virgin olive oil. Once the oil is heated, add the eggplant and garlic. Cook for 10 minutes. Stir occasionally. After 10 minutes, add the tomatoes, basil, and salt and pepper. Cook for an additional 20 minutes or until the mixture thickens. Fill a large pot with 1 gallon of salted cold water. Bring it to a boil. Once the water reaches a full boil, add the spaghetti and cook until al dente (chewy). Drain the spaghetti and add it to the sauce. Stir together and add the mozzarella cheese. Serve.

Cook's Tip: You can substitute low-fat ricotta cheese for the mozzarella cheese; you can also use penne, rigatoni, or any other pasta shape you desire to vary the texture of the dish.

Red Sea–Style Fish

This recipe, created by Kyle Shaddix, a registered dietitian and chef, is loaded with healthful fats. The simple flavors from the fresh tomato and onions are wonderful combinations with the classic flavor principles of northeastern Africa: garlic, cumin, and mint.

6 6-ounce white fish fillets, such as striped bass
pepper
1 teaspoon ground cumin
2 teaspoons fresh mint leaves, finely minced
1 tomato, diced
1 onion, cut into strips
1 clove garlic, minced
2 teaspoons extra-virgin olive oil
juice from 1 lemon

Total preparation and cooking time: **30** minutes

Makes 6 servings.

Nutrition information per serving:
Calories: 200
Fat: 6 g
Saturated fat: 1 g
Cholesterol: 135 mg
Sodium: 120 mg
Carbohydrate: 4 g
Fiber: 1 g
Sugar: 2 g
Protein: 31 g

Preheat oven to 400 degrees F. Place the fish fillets in a 9 by 11-inch pan lined with aluminum foil, leaving enough foil on the edges to cover the fish. Sprinkle the fish lightly with pepper to taste and lay it skin side down (if there is a skin side) on the foil. Sprinkle the cumin and mint leaves on the fish. Spread the tomatoes, onions, and garlic evenly over the fish and drizzle with the olive oil and lemon juice. Tightly seal the edges of the foil so the fish is airtight. Bake in the oven for 20 minutes until the fish flakes easily (place a fork into the thickest part of the fish and twist gently).

Cook's Tip: This recipe can also be made with codfish. It goes well with whole-wheat couscous and a green salad.

Roasted Tomatoes with Shrimp and Feta

This recipe from my dear friend Cindy Jennes is easy to prepare and very flavorful. It works well whether you're making dinner for company or just your own family.

5 large tomatoes, cut in eighths
3 tablespoons olive oil
3 tablespoons minced garlic
¾ teaspoon kosher salt
¾ teaspoon black pepper
1½ pounds medium shrimp, peeled and deveined
½ cup chopped fresh parsley
2 tablespoons lemon juice
1 cup feta cheese, crumbled

Total preparation and cooking time: 45 minutes

Makes 6 servings.

Nutrition information per serving:
Calories: 300
Fat: 15 g
Saturated fat: 5 g
Cholesterol: 245 mg
Sodium: 840 mg
Carbohydrate: 10 g
Fiber: 2 g
Sugar: 5 g
Protein: 28 g

Preheat oven to 450 degrees F. Place the tomatoes in a large baking dish (9 by 13 inches). Pour the olive oil and garlic over the tomatoes. Sprinkle with the salt and pepper and gently toss all the ingredients. Place on the top rack of the oven and roast for approximately 20 minutes. Remove the baking dish from the oven and stir in the shrimp, parsley, and lemon juice. Sprinkle with the feta. Place the baking dish back in the oven for another 10 to 15 minutes or until the shrimp are completely cooked.

Cook's Tip: To save fat and calories, you can use reduced-fat feta cheese without losing taste and texture. This dish is superb when served with warm crusty French or Italian bread.

Chipotle Lime Seared Salmon Fajitas

This is a tasty twist on traditional fajitas and a great way to incorporate healthful omega-3 fats into your diet.

1¼ pounds salmon filets cut into 1½-inch-wide
   slices
¼ cup lime juice
1 tablespoon Tabasco chipotle pepper sauce
2 tablespoons extra-virgin olive oil
1 tablespoon ground cumin
2 teaspoons chili powder
1 teaspoon salt
1 clove minced garlic
2 tablespoons chopped cilantro
nonstick cooking spray
1 cup sliced onion
1 red bell pepper cut into 1-inch strips
lime wedges
4 whole-wheat tortillas

Total preparation and cooking time: 1 hour

Makes 4 servings (4 fajitas).

Nutrition information per serving:
Calories: 300
Fat: 17 g
Saturated fat: 2.5 g
Cholesterol: 80 mg
Sodium: 690 mg
Carbohydrate: 8 g
Fiber: 2 g
Sugar: 3 g
Protein: 29 g

In a large bowl, combine the salmon with the lime juice, Tabasco chipotle pepper sauce, olive oil, cumin, chili powder, salt, garlic, and cilantro. Toss together well, cover, and refrigerate for 30 minutes. Spray a large nonstick skillet with the nonstick cooking spray and heat over medium heat. When the skillet is hot, add the onions and peppers and cook until softened, about 5 to 7 minutes. Remove the onions and peppers and add the seasoned salmon. Cook for 3 to 4 minutes until lightly brown. Then flip and continue cooking for an additional 3 to 4 minutes until firm inside. Combine with the peppers and onions. Serve wrapped in the whole-wheat tortillas you have warmed in the microwave for 10 to 15 seconds and garnish with the lime wedges.

Cook's Tip: This dish can also be served more traditionally alongside wild rice or pasta and a colorful vegetable medley.

Whole-Wheat Penne with Meatless Bolognese

This dish is sure to fool anyone who loves a rich meat sauce. Made with soy crumbles, the meatless bolognese is low in cholesterol and high in protein, and it has a delicious, creamy texture sure to please a variety of palates.

2 tablespoons olive oil
¾ cup finely chopped onion
2 cloves finely minced garlic
1 cup finely chopped carrots
½ cup finely chopped celery
½ teaspoon kosher salt
½ teaspoon ground pepper
¼ cup fresh chopped parsley
1 teaspoon oregano
6 ounces soy crumbles (about 2 cups)
1 28-ounce can whole peeled plum tomatoes, crushed
1 6-ounce can tomato paste
2 cups water
1 bay leaf
¼ cup fat-free half and half
1 pound whole-wheat penne pasta
6 tablespoons parmesan cheese, grated

Total preparation and cooking time: 2 hours and 20 minutes

Makes 6 servings.

Nutrition information per serving:
Calories: 410
Fat: 12 g
Saturated fat: 1.5 g
Cholesterol: 5 mg
Sodium: 1,010 mg
Carbohydrate: 62 g
Fiber: 11 g
Sugar: 9 g
Protein: 20 g

In a large pot over medium heat, heat the olive oil. Sauté the onions, garlic, carrots, and celery for 6 to 7 minutes until softened and lightly browned. Add the salt, pepper, parsley, oregano, and soy crumbles, and cook an additional 5 minutes until well combined. Add the plum tomatoes, tomato paste, water, and bay leaf, and bring to a boil, stirring occasionally. Reduce the heat to low and simmer for 1 hour and 45 minutes. Stir in the half and half and cook for an additional 5 minutes. Cook the pasta according to the package directions. Drain

Whole-Wheat Penne with Meatless Bolognese *(continued)*

and toss with the sauce. Sprinkle with the parmesan cheese.

Cook's Tip: To save on sodium, you can choose low-sodium tomato paste and/or delete the added salt, which does not significantly alter the taste of the sauce, especially if you tend to like your food more bland.

Eli's Chicken Meatballs and Spaghetti

These meatballs are among my younger son Eli's favorite foods. From an early age, he has eaten these meatballs, created by his caregiver, Linda, at least two nights each week. He loves to dip them in grated parmesan cheese and have them on top of whole-wheat macaroni. Because he loves this recipe so much, I decided to steal it from my last book, So What Can I Eat?! *(Wiley, 2006) so families everywhere can enjoy it.*

16 ounces lean ground chicken breast
¼ cup bread crumbs, seasoned
¼ cup finely chopped red onion
1 clove minced garlic
2 tablespoons fresh parsley
¼ teaspoon kosher salt
¼ teaspoon pepper
2 cups tomato sauce (jarred)
8 ounces (½ box) thin spaghetti, cooked
¼ cup grated parmesan cheese

Total preparation and cooking time: 45 minutes

Makes 4 servings.

Nutrition information per serving:
Calories: 420
Fat: 4.5 g
Saturated fat: 1.5 g
Cholesterol: 70 mg
Sodium: 990 mg
Carbohydrate: 58 g
Fiber: 4 g
Sugar: 8 g
Protein: 39 g

In a large bowl, combine the chicken with the bread crumbs, red onion, garlic, parsley, salt, and pepper until ingredients are evenly distributed. Form into 12 meatballs. Set a large pan on medium to high heat. Add the tomato sauce and bring to a boil. When the sauce is boiling, put the meatballs in, lower the heat, and cover. Cook for 10 to 15 minutes. Add to the cooked thin spaghetti, top with 1 tablespoon of parmesan cheese, and serve.

Cook's Tip: This recipe is admittedly high in sodium, but you can lower the sodium content substantially (without altering the flavor too much) if you use low-sodium tomato sauce and/or skip the salt. These meatballs can also be sliced and served cold on whole-grain bread for lunch the next day.

Penne with Shrimp and Broccoli Rabe

This rustic pasta dish is a perfect way to get some healthful vegetables, whole grains, and lean protein all in one tasty meal.

½ pound whole-wheat penne pasta
1 pound broccoli rabe, stems removed and chopped
2 tablespoons extra-virgin olive oil
2 cloves chopped garlic
¾ teaspoon kosher salt
½ pound large shrimp, peeled and deveined
¼ teaspoon crushed red pepper
1 cup tomato, chopped
2 tablespoons fresh chopped basil

Total preparation and cooking time: 30 minutes

Makes 4 servings.

Nutrition information per serving:
Calories: 370
Fat: 9 g
Saturated fat: 1.5 g
Cholesterol: 85 mg
Sodium: 560 mg
Carbohydrate: 51 g
Fiber: 5 g
Sugar: 3 g
Protein: 24 g

Cook the pasta according to the package directions. During the last 5 minutes of cooking, add the broccoli rabe to the pasta pot and cook for the remaining 5 minutes. Drain, but reserve ½ cup of the pasta water and set aside. Heat a large skillet with the olive oil on medium heat. Add the garlic and salt and allow the garlic to brown for about 1 to 2 minutes. Add the shrimp and crushed red pepper, and cook for an additional 3 to 4 minutes. Add ½ cup of the reserved pasta water and cook an additional 1 to 2 minutes. Add the pasta and broccoli rabe and toss together adding the tomato and basil. Toss all the ingredients together until well incorporated. Serve.

Cook's Tip: You can substitute broccoli florets for the broccoli rabe if desired. You can use grated parmesan cheese as a garnish.

One-Pot Vegetable Beef Chili

This dish is so tasty and a great way to sneak some extra fiber into a meal.

2 15½-ounce cans kidney beans
1 15½-ounce can black beans (low sodium)
6 ounces ground sirloin
1 28-ounce can crushed tomatoes
¼ cup tomato paste
½ package (6 ounces) soy crumbles
½ cup chopped red onion
2 cloves minced garlic
1 cup corn kernels
1 cup chopped red bell pepper
1 tablespoon jalapeño pepper, finely diced
1 1¼-ounce package low-sodium chili seasoning mix
½ cup chopped cilantro

Total preparation and cooking time: 4 hours and 15 minutes

Makes 8 servings.

Nutrition information per serving:

Calories: 360
Fat: 6 g
Saturated fat: 0 g
Cholesterol: 10 mg
Sodium: 910 mg
Carbohydrate: 53 g
Fiber: 18 g
Sugar: 5 g
Protein: 25 g

Place all ingredients in a 4-quart slow cooker. Stir a few times to make sure all the ingredients are combined. Cover and cook on high for 4 hours.

Cook's Tip: This chili tastes great alone or you can top it with some low-fat cheddar cheese and/or low-fat sour cream.

Cheesy Chicken Fajitas

This is one of my signature dishes that all my boys (including my husband) love. It's so easy to prepare, with few ingredients yet a lot of flavor.

1 pound chicken breast, skinless and boneless
4 teaspoons light teriyaki sauce, low sodium
1 cup low-sodium tomato sauce
2 tablespoons canola oil
1 cup low-fat shredded cheddar cheese
4 flour tortillas, 2 ounces each

Total preparation and cooking time: 30 minutes (including 10 minutes to marinate)

Makes 4 servings.

Nutrition information per serving:
Calories: 420
Fat: 14 g
Saturated fat: 3 g
Cholesterol: 70 mg
Sodium: 570 mg
Carbohydrate: 33 g
Fiber: 3 g
Protein: 38 g

Cut the chicken breast into thin strips. Place in a bowl. Add the teriyaki sauce and tomato sauce and combine so they cover all the chicken strips evenly. Let the chicken marinate for 10 minutes. Heat a large skillet on medium heat with 2 tablespoons of canola oil. When the oil is hot, add the chicken and sauté for about 5 minutes, stirring frequently. Then add the cheese and continue to stir for about 5 more minutes. When the chicken is thoroughly cooked, place in a bowl lined with a paper towel and blot to remove excess oil. Add the chicken mixture to the flour tortillas and roll into a wrap. Warm each fajita in the microwave for about 50 seconds each. Allow to cool for 1 minute, and then serve cut up for the kids (or serve whole).

Cook's Tip: These taste delicious, especially when served with salsa or reduced-fat sour cream. To serve as an appetizer, divide the fajitas into triangles. To save time (and oil), you can grill the chicken. This recipe can also be made with a lean meat like flank steak.

Spinach and Sausage Lasagna

My family loves lasagna, but not all the fat and calories. This healthier version is so scrumptious, it's hard to resist having seconds. This recipe makes 12 servings, so make it and freeze in shallow containers for a quick last-minute meal.

1 pound lean turkey or chicken sausage, casing removed
¾ cup chopped onion
1 clove minced garlic
1 tablespoon chopped fresh sage or 1 teaspoon dried
3 cups low-fat ricotta cheese
1 10-ounce package frozen chopped spinach, thawed and squeezed dry
3 tablespoons grated parmesan cheese
2 egg whites
1 29-ounce can low-sodium tomato sauce
1½ cups reduced-fat shredded mozzarella cheese
9 oven-ready lasagna noodles
nonstick cooking spray

Total cooking and preparation time: 1 hour and 30 minutes

Makes 12 servings.

Nutrition information per serving:
Calories: 340
Fat: 10 g
Saturated fat: 4.5 g
Cholesterol: 55 mg
Sodium: 440 mg
Carbohydrate: 39 g
Fiber: 3 g
Sugar: 6 g
Protein: 23 g

Preheat oven to 375 degrees F. Heat a nonstick skillet over medium heat, add the sausage, and cook for 5 minutes until lightly brown. Add the onions, garlic, and sage, and cook an additional 10 minutes until the sausage is no longer pink. In a blender or food processor, combine the ricotta with the spinach, parmesan cheese, and egg whites, and set aside. Spread 1 cup of the tomato sauce on the bottom of a 13 by 9-inch baking dish, and top with 3 strips of noodles. Top the noodles with ½ of the spinach mixture, ½ of the sausage mixture, ½ cup of the shredded cheese, and 1½ cups of the tomato sauce. Repeat the layering with 3 more noodles, the remaining cheese mixture, sausage, ½ cup shredded cheese and 1½ cups sauce. Top with the remaining noodles, sauce, and ½ cup shredded cheese. Spray a sheet of aluminum foil with the nonstick cooking spray and cover the lasagna.

Spinach and Sausage Lasagna *(continued)*

Bake for 45 minutes. Remove the foil and cook
for an additional 5 to 10 minutes until the cheese
is melted and bubbly. Cool 10 minutes before
serving.

Cook's Tip: You can add shredded carrots or
any other vegetables you desire for added flavor,
color, and nutrients.

Side Dishes

Couscous with Asparagus, Orange, and Mint

This dish serves as a tangy, tasty way to get some green vegetables into your diet with great texture and flavor.

1 box instant couscous (10 ounces)
1 tablespoon extra-virgin olive oil
1 cup chopped fresh asparagus (about ½ pound)
¼ cup diced scallion
½ teaspoon kosher salt
½ teaspoon fresh ground pepper
½ cup low-sodium, fat-free chicken broth
3 tablespoons fresh squeezed orange juice
2 teaspoons orange zest
⅓ cup chopped fresh mint
¾ cup orange segments (about 1 medium orange)

Total preparation and cooking time: 20 minutes

Makes 6 servings.

Nutrition information per serving:
Calories: 220
Fat: 3.5 g
Saturated fat: 1 g
Cholesterol: 0 mg
Sodium: 260 mg
Carbohydrate: 41 g
Fiber: 4 g
Sugar: 3 g
Protein: 8 g

Prepare the couscous according to the package instructions. Set aside. Heat the olive oil in a medium sauté pan over medium heat. Sauté the asparagus with the scallions, salt, and pepper for 5 minutes or until tender. Add the chicken broth, orange juice, and zest, and cook an additional 2 to 3 minutes. Add the asparagus mixture to the couscous and toss together well, adding the mint and orange segments. Transfer to a platter and serve cold.

Cook's Tip: This dish tastes great alongside chicken or fish.

Baked Yukon-Gold Mustard Fries

Who doesn't love French fries? This is a trans fat–free alternative to your typical fast-food fries, one your kids (and you) are sure to love.

1½ pounds Yukon Gold potatoes cut into wedges, lengthwise
1 tablespoon canola oil
7 tablespoons whole-grain mustard
1 teaspoon Tabasco sauce
¼ teaspoon onion powder
¼ teaspoon garlic powder
½ teaspoon dried oregano
nonstick cooking spray
2 tablespoons honey
2 tablespoons chopped scallion

Total preparation and cooking time: 1 hour and 15 minutes

Makes 6 servings.

Nutrition information per serving:
Calories: 230
Fat: 8 g
Saturated fat: 1 g
Cholesterol: 0 mg
Sodium: 520 mg
Carbohydrate: 39 g
Fiber: 3 g
Sugar: 12 g
Protein: 4 g

Preheat oven to 375 degrees F. In a medium bowl, toss the potatoes with the canola oil, 3 tablespoons of the mustard, the Tabasco sauce, onion powder, garlic powder, and oregano until well coated. Spray a roasting pan with the nonstick cooking spray. Spread the potatoes on the pan and cook for 25 minutes. Then turn the potatoes and cook for an additional 25 to 30 minutes until golden and crisp. While potatoes are cooking, in a small bowl mix together the honey, 4 tablespoons of the mustard, and the scallions. Set aside until ready to serve.

Cook's Tip: You can use honey mustard instead of the traditional ketchup as a dip. Do not give honey to children under the age of one because of the risk of botulism.

Sweet and Tangy Asparagus

This dish gives a zesty twist to asparagus with a sweet citrus flavor.
It's so good, it may even encourage your kids to eat their vegetables.

½ teaspoon kosher salt
1 pound asparagus, stemmed
2 tablespoons orange juice
1 tablespoon honey
1 tablespoon balsamic vinegar
2 tablespoons extra-virgin olive oil
½ teaspoon orange zest
¼ cup orange segments, cut in thirds
fresh ground pepper

Total cooking and preparation time: 20 minutes

Makes 6 servings.

Nutrition information per serving:
Calories: 80
Fat: 5 g
Saturated fat: 0.5 g
Cholesterol: 0 mg
Sodium: 200 mg
Carbohydrate: 8 g
Fiber: 2 g
Sugar: 6 g
Protein: 2 g

Fill a medium pan halfway with water and ¼ teaspoon of the kosher salt, cover, and bring to a boil. Add the asparagus and cover for about 3 to 5 minutes until tender. Drain and rinse with cold water to chill. Set aside. In a medium bowl, whisk the orange juice, honey, vinegar, olive oil, the remaining ¼ teaspoon of salt, and the orange zest. Add the orange segments and toss in the asparagus. Season to taste with the pepper. Serve cold.

Cook's Tip: This dish can be made ahead and kept covered in the refrigerator until ready to serve. It goes well with lean red meat, chicken, or fish.

Sweets and Treats

Incredibly Good Chocolate Chip Walnut Cookies

These cookies are so delicious, it's hard to believe they're low-fat.

⅓ cup brown sugar
⅓ cup white sugar
2 tablespoons melted trans fat–free margarine
3 teaspoons vanilla extract
2 egg whites
1¼ cups all-purpose flour
1 teaspoon baking soda
½ teaspoon salt
⅓ cup milk chocolate or semisweet chocolate chips
¼ cup chopped walnuts
nonstick cooking spray

Total preparation and cooking time: 45 minutes

Makes 24 cookies (1 cookie per serving).

Nutrition information per serving:
Calories: 80
Fat: 2.5 g
Saturated fat: 1 g
Cholesterol: 0 mg
Sodium: 115 mg
Carbohydrate: 12 g
Fiber: 0 g
Sugar: 7 g
Protein: 1 g

Preheat oven to 350 degrees F. Using an electric mixer at medium speed, combine the brown sugar, white sugar, melted margarine, and vanilla until well blended (about 3 minutes). Add the egg whites and beat for an additional 2 minutes. Lower the speed and slowly add the flour, baking soda, and salt, and beat an additional 2 to 3 minutes. Scrape the bowl so that all the flour gets incorporated. Stir in the chocolate chips and walnuts. Prepare 2 cookie sheets with the nonstick cooking spray. Drop approximately 1 tablespoon of cookie dough for each cookie. Bake for 10 to 12 minutes until lightly golden. Cool on a rack for 10 minutes or longer before serving.

Super Strawberry Smoothie

This flavorful, easy-to-make smoothie makes a great on-the-go snack that helps you incorporate fiber-rich strawberries and low-fat yogurt, a great source of calcium. Wheat germ adds additional fiber, folic acid, and vitamin E as well.

1 cup strawberries cut in half, washed and stems
  removed
½ cup fat-free vanilla yogurt
2 tablespoons honey crunch wheat germ
1 tablespoon honey
2 tablespoons skim milk
4 ice cubes

Place all the ingredients in a blender and blend for 2 to 3 minutes until thick and smooth. Serve cold, and garnish with an extra strawberry if desired.

Cook's Tip: You can use orange juice to replace skim milk for a more tangy smoothie. You can also divide to make three ½-cup servings to provide a quick energy boost with fewer calories. Do not give honey to children under the age of one because of the risk of botulism.

Total preparation and cooking time: 10 minutes

Makes 1 serving (1½ cups).

Nutrition information per serving:
Calories: 300
Fat: 2 g
Saturated fat: 0 g
Cholesterol: 5 mg
Sodium: 105 mg
Carbohydrate: 63 g
Fiber: 5 g
Sugar: 4 g
Protein: 13 g

Tropical Oatmeal Raisin Cookies

These cookies are so moist, fruity and chewy, they're hard to resist.
Thank goodness they're low in fat!

nonstick cooking spray
1½ cups old-fashioned rolled oats
1¼ cups all-purpose flour
¼ teaspoon ground cinnamon
½ teaspoon baking soda
¼ teaspoon salt
¾ cup dark brown sugar
¼ cup honey
2 egg whites
1 teaspoon vanilla extract
¼ teaspoon coconut extract
½ cup dried fruit bits
1 tablespoon chopped crystallized ginger
2 tablespoons shredded coconut

Total preparation and
cooking time: 1 hour

Makes 28 cookies (1
cookie per serving).

Nutrition information
per serving:
Calories: 80
Fat: 0.5 g
Saturated fat: 0 g
Cholesterol: 0 mg
Sodium: 50 mg
Carbohydrate: 18 g
Fiber: 1 g
Sugar: 10 g
Protein: 2 g

Preheat oven to 325 degrees F. Spray 2 cookie
sheets with the nonstick cooking spray, and set
them aside. In a bowl, combine the oats, flour,
cinnamon, baking soda, and salt, and set aside. In
an electric mixer, beat the sugar, honey, egg whites,
vanilla, and coconut extract until smooth. Add
half of the oat mixture and mix again. Then add
the remaining oat mixture, fruit bits, ginger, and
shredded coconut until well combined. Drop 1
heaping tablespoon of cookie dough 2 inches
apart on the cookie sheets to form each cookie.
Bake 10 to 12 minutes or until golden. Let cool
5 minutes. Transfer cookies to a cooling rack, and
cool completely.

Banana Nut Loaf Cake

What a delicious way to incorporate healthful nuts and fiber-rich fruit into your diet! The whole-wheat flour and wheat germ also provide additional fiber to help you meet your daily quota.

1 cup bran flakes cereal
1 cup low-fat milk
½ cup whole-wheat flour
½ cup all-purpose flour
1 teaspoon baking soda
½ cup sugar
½ cup golden raisins
½ cup chopped walnuts
½ cup wheat germ
3 bananas, mashed
2 eggs
2 tablespoons powdered sugar

Total preparation and cooking time: 2 hours and 30 minutes

Makes 10 servings.

Nutrition information per serving:
Calories: 220
Fat: 6 g
Saturated fat: 1 g
Cholesterol: 45 mg
Sodium: 180 mg
Carbohydrate: 39 g
Fiber: 4 g
Sugar: 20 g
Protein: 7 g

Preheat oven to 350 degrees F. Place the bran flakes in a small bowl, cover with the milk, and allow to stand for 10 to 15 minutes. In a large bowl, combine the flour, baking soda, sugar, raisins, walnuts, and wheat germ. Stir well. Mash the bananas thoroughly, break in the eggs, and stir to combine. Add the banana mixture and soaked bran flakes to the dry ingredients. Mix well. Pour the mixture into a greased loaf pan, and bake for approximately 1 hour or until a toothpick inserted in the center comes out clean. Turn onto a cooling rack and let stand for at least 15 minutes before slicing. Sprinkle with the powdered sugar.

Cook's Tip: You can freeze this cake in slices and defrost one for a midday snack. This can also be a great complement to string cheese as a quick on-the-go breakfast as you head out the door.

Quick and Easy Low-Fat Pumpkin Pie

Whether it's for a holiday or special event, or simply a tasty dessert for any time, this recipe offers a lot of flavor without too much fat or sugar.

2 egg whites
⅔ cup light brown sugar
1 15-ounce can pumpkin purée
1 12-ounce can nonfat evaporated milk
1 teaspoon ground cinnamon
¼ teaspoon ground nutmeg
½ teaspoon ground ginger
¼ teaspoon ground cloves
1 9-inch frozen deep-dish pie shell

Total preparation and cooking time: 1 hour and 20 minutes (4 hours to cool)

Makes 12 servings (slices).

Nutrition information per serving:
Calories: 120
Fat: 3.5 g
Saturated fat: 1.5 g
Cholesterol: 5 mg
Sodium: 100 mg
Carbohydrate: 18 g
Fiber: 2 g
Sugar: 10 g
Protein: 4 g

Preheat oven to 400 degrees F. In a large bowl, whisk the egg whites with the sugar until smooth. Add the pumpkin purée, evaporated milk, cinnamon, nutmeg, ginger, and cloves until well combined. Fill the pie shell and place it on a baking sheet. Bake for 20 minutes, reduce heat to 350 degrees F, and bake for an additional 40 to 45 minutes until set. Allow to cool completely (about 4 hours). Serve.

Chips and Dips

Beany Nachos

Perfect for those sports-filled Sundays, this is a snack that everyone will enjoy.

1 16-ounce can fat-free/nonfat refried beans
1 teaspoon ground cumin
1 tablespoon lime juice
1 cup chopped plum tomatoes
2 tablespoons chopped jalapeño peppers
2 tablespoons chopped red onion
1 tablespoon Tabasco sauce
¼ cup chopped fresh cilantro
8 ounces baked tortilla chips
1 cup reduced-fat shredded cheddar cheese
2 tablespoons fat-free (or nonfat) sour cream

Total cooking and preparation time: 20 minutes.

Makes 6 servings.

Nutrition information per serving:
Calories: 230
Fat: 2 g
Saturated fat: 0 g
Cholesterol: 0 mg
Sodium: 720 mg
Carbohydrate: 45 g
Fiber: 7 g
Sugar: 2 g
Protein: 8 g

Preheat oven to 375 degrees F. In a bowl, combine the refried beans with the cumin and lime juice, and set aside. In a separate bowl, combine the tomatoes, jalapeño peppers, red onion, Tabasco sauce, and 2 tablespoons of the cilantro, and set aside. Spread the bottom of an ovenproof serving platter with a single layer of the chips, top with ½ of the bean mixture, ½ the tomato mixture, and ½ cup of the shredded cheese. Top with the remaining chips, bean, and tomato mixture, and sprinkle with the remaining cheese. Bake until heated through and the cheese is melted and bubbly, about 8 to 10 minutes. Garnish with the sour cream and remaining chopped cilantro.

> **Cook's Tip:** This dip also tastes great spread on a warm flour tortilla or as a dip for raw vegetables.

Smoky Chipotle and Red Pepper Dip

This is a great crowd-pleasing dip.

¼ cup sliced almonds
2 cloves garlic
2 tablespoons chopped scallion
½ cup roasted red peppers (jarred)
¼ teaspoon salt
¼ teaspoon ground chipotle pepper
¼ cup nonfat sour cream
2 teaspoons Tabasco chipotle pepper sauce

Total preparation and cooking time: 25 minutes

Makes 6 servings.

Nutrition information per serving:

Calories: 60
Fat: 2 g
Saturated fat: 0 g
Cholesterol: 0 mg
Sodium: 360 mg
Carbohydrate: 7 g
Fiber: 1 g
Sugar: 1 g
Protein: 2 g

Process the almonds in a food processor until ground fine. Add the garlic, scallion, red peppers, salt, and chipotle pepper, and process until well blended. Transfer to a bowl and fold in the sour cream and Tabasco chipotle pepper sauce until smooth.

Cook's Tip: Serve with baked tortilla chips or cut-up vegetables. This dip tastes even better if it is made ahead of time and chilled, and then served.

Delicious Shrimp Dip

This elegant dip is easy to make and tastes fresh and light. It's also an excellent way to incorporate fish in your diet.

1 8-ounce package Neufchâtel cream cheese, at room temperature
½ cup reduced-fat sour cream
¼ cup chopped scallions
¼ cup chopped dill
2 tablespoons chopped fresh parsley
1 tablespoon chopped fresh tarragon
2 teaspoons lemon zest
¼ teaspoon salt
1 teaspoon Tabasco sauce
2 cups chopped cooked shrimp

Total cooking and preparation time: 1 hour and 15 minutes

Makes 10 servings.

Nutrition information per serving:
Calories: 130
Fat: 7 g
Saturated fat: 4.5 g
Cholesterol: 75 mg
Sodium: 260 mg
Carbohydrate: 7 g
Fiber: 3 g
Sugar: 4 g
Protein: 10 g

Beat the cream cheese and the sour cream with an electric mixer until smooth. Add the scallions, dill, parsley, tarragon, lemon zest, salt, and Tabasco sauce until well combined. Stir in the shrimp and continue beating another 2 minutes until all ingredients are incorporated. Refrigerate for 1 hour and serve.

Cook's Tip: Serve with red bell pepper strips, baby carrots, celery sticks, endive, or whole-grain crackers.

Anselma's Famous Guacamole

Avocados are a rich source of vitamin E, potassium, and fiber. Even though they contain a lot of fat, it's mostly heart-healthy monoun-saturated fat. My dear friend Anselma, also a registered dietitian, swears by this guacamole. Her young sons, Sebastian and Luca, have devoured it since they were toddlers and now love to have it as an after-school snack.

5 avocados
½ cup lime juice (approximate yield from 2 fresh 2-inch limes)
2 ripe tomatoes, chopped
1 small red onion, chopped
pinch of salt
1 tablespoon olive oil
½ teaspoon cumin

Total preparation and cooking time: 4 hours and 10 minutes

Makes 16 servings.

Nutrition information per serving:
Calories: 140
Fat: 12 g
Saturated fat: 1.5 g
Cholesterol: 0 mg
Sodium: 45 mg
Carbohydrate: 9 g
Fiber: 5 g
Sugar: 1 g
Protein: 2 g

Cut the avocados in half and remove the seeds. Scoop out the pulp from the avocados and mash in a large bowl. Add the lime juice, tomatoes, red onion, salt, olive oil, and cumin, and mash until completely blended. Let the mixture chill in the refrigerator for a few hours to allow the flavors to infuse. Serve.

Cook's Tip: You can buy avocados when they're a bit hard and let them ripen on your kitchen counter. This dip tastes great with baked tortilla chips, fresh vegetable slices, or baked whole-wheat pita bread cut into triangles.

APPENDIX A
Your Family's Genes

Your Family's Genetic Bodies					
Family Member	BMI Category	Body Shape	Waist Circumference	Frame Size[a]	Significant Medical History[b]

[a]*Frame size is applicable only to adults.*
[b]*Record any diseases or conditions you have now or have had in the past. See chapter 11 for more information.*

APPENDIX B
Body Mass Index

Body mass index (BMI) measures your weight in relation to your height. It is a useful tool to use to estimate how much body fat you have. The adults in your family can calculate their own BMI values and plot such values in the chart in appendix A. Your pediatrician can determine and assess your child's BMI, which will change from year to year as he or she grows.

Adults

On pages 230 and 231 is a chart to help you and other family members twenty years of age or older determine your individual body mass index (BMI). Find your height in the left-hand column. Then move across in the same row to the number closest to your weight. The number at the top of that column is your BMI. Check the word above your BMI to see whether your body weight is considered normal, overweight, or obese. When you determine your BMI, note in the chart in appendix A the category into which you fall.

BMI for Children

In children and teens, BMI is used to assess underweight, overweight, and the risk for overweight. Children's body fatness changes over the years as they grow. Also, girls and boys differ in their body fatness as they mature. This is why BMI for children, also referred to as BMI-for-age, is gender and age specific. For all children, it's best to see a pediatrician who can assess how they're growing in terms of weight and height. The pediatrician will use growth charts, including the recently released World Health Organization Child Growth Standards that include standardized BMI charts for infants to age five to assess healthy weight in children. See www.who.int/childgrowth/standards/en/.

Body Mass Index																	
	Normal						Overweight					Obese					
BMI	19	20	21	22	23	24	25	26	27	28	29	30	31	32	33	34	35	36
Height (inches)	Body Weight (pounds)																
58	91	96	100	105	110	115	119	124	129	134	138	143	148	153	158	162	167	172
59	94	99	104	109	114	119	124	128	133	138	143	148	153	158	163	168	173	178
60	97	102	107	112	118	123	128	133	138	143	148	153	158	163	168	174	179	184
61	100	106	111	116	122	127	132	137	143	148	153	158	164	169	174	180	185	190
62	104	109	115	120	126	131	136	142	147	153	158	164	169	175	180	186	191	196
63	107	113	118	124	130	135	141	146	152	158	163	169	175	180	186	191	197	203
64	110	116	122	128	134	140	145	151	157	163	169	174	180	186	192	197	204	209
65	114	120	126	132	138	144	150	156	162	168	174	180	186	192	198	204	210	216
66	118	124	130	136	142	148	155	161	167	173	179	186	192	198	204	210	216	223
67	121	127	134	140	146	153	159	166	172	178	185	191	198	204	211	217	223	230
68	125	131	138	144	151	158	164	171	177	184	190	197	203	210	216	223	230	236
69	128	135	142	149	155	162	169	176	182	189	196	203	209	216	223	230	236	243
70	132	139	146	153	160	167	174	181	188	195	202	209	216	222	229	236	243	250
71	136	143	150	157	165	172	179	186	193	200	208	215	222	229	236	243	250	257
72	140	147	154	162	169	177	184	191	199	206	213	221	228	235	242	250	258	265
73	144	151	159	166	174	182	189	197	204	212	219	227	235	242	250	257	265	272
74	148	155	163	171	179	186	194	202	210	218	225	233	241	249	256	264	272	280
75	152	160	168	176	184	192	200	208	216	224	232	240	248	256	264	272	279	287
76	156	164	172	180	189	197	205	213	221	230	238	246	254	263	271	279	287	295

Body Mass Index																		
	Obese			Extreme Obesity														
BMI	37	38	39	40	41	42	43	44	45	46	47	48	49	50	51	52	53	54
Height (inches)	Body Weight (pounds)																	
58	177	181	186	191	196	201	205	210	215	220	224	229	234	239	244	248	253	258
59	183	188	193	198	203	208	212	217	222	227	232	237	242	247	252	257	262	267
60	189	194	199	204	209	215	220	225	230	235	240	245	250	255	261	266	271	276
61	195	201	206	211	217	222	227	232	238	243	248	254	259	264	269	275	280	285
62	202	207	213	218	224	229	235	240	246	251	256	262	267	273	278	284	289	295
63	208	214	220	225	231	237	242	248	254	259	265	270	278	282	287	293	299	304
64	215	221	227	232	238	244	250	256	262	267	273	279	285	291	296	302	308	314
65	222	228	234	240	246	252	258	264	270	276	282	288	294	300	306	312	318	324
66	229	235	241	247	253	260	266	272	278	284	291	297	303	309	315	322	328	334
67	236	242	249	255	261	268	274	280	287	293	299	306	312	319	325	331	338	344
68	243	249	256	262	269	276	282	289	295	302	308	315	322	328	335	341	348	354
69	250	257	263	270	277	284	291	297	304	311	318	324	331	338	345	351	358	365
70	257	264	271	278	285	292	299	306	313	320	327	334	341	348	355	362	369	376
71	265	272	279	286	293	301	308	315	322	329	338	343	351	358	365	372	379	386
72	272	279	287	294	302	309	316	324	331	338	346	353	361	368	375	383	390	397
73	280	288	295	302	310	318	325	333	340	348	355	363	371	378	386	393	401	408
74	287	295	303	311	319	326	334	342	350	358	365	373	381	389	396	404	412	420
75	295	303	311	319	327	335	343	351	359	367	375	383	391	399	407	415	423	431
76	304	312	320	328	336	344	353	361	369	377	385	394	402	410	418	426	435	443

Source: Adapted from Clinical Guidelines on the Identification, Evaluation, and Treatment of Overweight and Obesity in Adults: The Evidence Report, *(National Institutes of Health, September 1998).*

APPENDIX C
Frame Size

To determine your body frame size, measure your wrist (in inches) with a flat tape measure to determine wrist circumference. Plot your height and wrist measurements as shown here to determine if you have a small, medium, or large frame. You can photocopy this and complete it for all family members. Record your frame size in the chart in appendix A. This measurement is appropriate only for use in adults.

Your height: _____ feet ____ inches

Your wrist circumference: _____ inches

Women

You have a small frame if:

- Your height is less than 5'2" and wrist measurement is less than 5.5".
- Your height is 5'2" to 5'5" and wrist measurement is 5.5" to less than 6.0".
- Your height is more than 5'5" and wrist measurement is 6.0" to less than 6.25".

You have a medium frame if:

- Your height is less than 5'2" and wrist measurement is 5.5" to 5.75".
- Your height is 5'2" to 5'5" and wrist measurement is 6.0" to 6.25".
- Your height is more than 5'5" and wrist measurement is 6.25" to 6.5".

You have a large frame if:

- Your height is less than 5'2" and wrist measurement is more than 5.75".
- Your height is 5'2" to 5'5" and wrist measurement is more than 6.25".
- Your height is more than 5'5" and wrist measurement is more than 6.5".

Males

- You have a small frame if your height is more than 5'5" and wrist measurement is 5.5" to 6.5".
- You have a medium frame if your height is more than 5'5" and wrist measurement is 6.5" to 7.5".
- You have a large frame if your height is more than 5'5" and wrist measurement is more than 7.5".

APPENDIX D
Food Sources of Key Nutrients

Following is a list of key nutrients, including vitamins, minerals, and fiber, you and your family need. The amounts needed by adults are provided. Children's needs are likely to be met if they follow an appropriate meal plan for their age and gender as described in chapter 10.

Vitamin A

Food sources are ranked by micrograms (µg) retinol activity equivalents (RAEs) of vitamin A per standard amount. Women need 700 micrograms per day (1,300 milligrams per day during lactation) and men need 900 micrograms per day.

Food, Standard Amount	Vitamin A (µg)
Carrot juice, ¾ cup	1,692
Sweet potato with peel, baked, 1 medium	1,096
Pumpkin, canned, ½ cup	953
Carrots, cooked from fresh, ½ cup	671
Spinach, cooked from frozen, ½ cup	573
Collards, cooked from frozen, ½ cup	489
Kale, cooked from frozen, ½ cup	478
Mixed vegetables, canned, ½ cup	474
Turnip greens, cooked from frozen, ½ cup	441
Instant cooked cereals, fortified, prepared, 1 packet	285–376
Various ready-to-eat cereals, with added vitamin A, approximately 1 ounce	180–376
Carrot, raw, 1 small	301
Beet greens, cooked, ½ cup	276

Food, Standard Amount	Vitamin A (µg)
Winter squash, cooked, ½ cup	268
Dandelion greens, cooked, ½ cup	260
Cantaloupe, raw, ¼ medium melon	233
Mustard greens, cooked, ½ cup	221
Pickled herring, 3 ounces	219
Red sweet pepper, cooked, ½ cup	186
Chinese cabbage, cooked, ½ cup	180

Source: Nutrient values from the Agricultural Research Service (ARS) Nutrient Database for Standard Reference, Release 17. Foods are from the ARS single nutrient reports, sorted in descending order by nutrient content in terms of common household measures. Food items and weights in the single nutrient reports are adapted from those in the 2002 revision of USDA Home and Garden Bulletin no. 72, "Nutritive Value of Foods." Mixed dishes and multiple preparations of the same food item are omitted from this table.

Vitamin C

Food sources are ranked by milligrams of vitamin C per standard amount. Women need 75 milligrams per day (120 milligrams per day when lactating), and men need 90 milligrams per day.

Food, Standard Amount	Vitamin C (mg)
Guava, raw, ½ cup	188
Red sweet pepper, raw, ½ cup	142
Red sweet pepper, cooked, ½ cup	116
Kiwifruit, 1 medium	70
Orange, raw, 1 medium	70
Orange juice, ¾ cup	61–93
Green pepper, sweet, raw, ½ cup	60
Green pepper, sweet, cooked, ½ cup	51
Grapefruit juice, ¾ cup	50–70
Vegetable juice cocktail, ¾ cup	50
Strawberries, raw, ½ cup	49
Brussels sprouts, cooked, ½ cup	48
Cantaloupe, ¼ medium	47
Papaya, raw, ¼ medium	47
Kohlrabi, cooked, ½ cup	45
Broccoli, raw, ½ cup	39

Food, Standard Amount	Vitamin C (mg)
Edible peapods, cooked, ½ cup	38
Broccoli, cooked, ½ cup	37
Sweet potato, canned, ½ cup	34
Tomato juice, ¾ cup	33
Cauliflower, cooked, ½ cup	28
Pineapple, raw, ½ cup	28
Kale, cooked, ½ cup	27
Mango, ½ cup	23

Source: Nutrient values from the Agricultural Research Service (ARS) Nutrient Database for Standard Reference, Release 17. Foods are from the ARS single nutrient reports, sorted in descending order by nutrient content in terms of common household measures. Food items and weights in the single nutrient reports are adapted from those in the 2002 revision of USDA Home and Garden Bulletin no. 72, "Nutritive Value of Foods". Mixed dishes and multiple preparations of the same food item are omitted from this table.

Vitamin D

Food sources are ranked by international units (IU) of vitamin D per standard amount. Adults fifty and under need 200 IU per day, and those fifty-one to seventy years need 400 IU per day. Needs increase to 600 IU per day for those over the age of seventy.

Food, Standard Amount	Vitamin D (IU)
Cod liver oil, 1 tablespoon	1,360
Salmon, cooked, 3 ½ ounces	360
Mackerel, cooked, 3 ½ ounces	345
Sardines, canned in oil, drained, 1¾ ounces	250
Tuna fish, canned in oil, 3 ounces	200
Milk, nonfat, reduced fat, and whole, vitamin D fortified, 1 cup	98
Margarine, fortified, 1 tablespoon	60
Pudding, prepared from mix and made with vitamin D fortified milk, ½ cup	50
Ready-to-eat cereals fortified with 10 percent of the daily value for vitamin D, ¾-cup to 1-cup servings (servings vary according to the brand)	40
Egg, 1 whole (vitamin D is found in egg yolk)	20
Liver, beef, cooked, 3 ½ ounces	15
Swiss cheese, 1 ounce	12

Source: Dietary Supplement Fact Sheet: Vitamin D, Office of Dietary Supplements, NIH Clinical Center, National Institutes of Health.

Vitamin E

Food sources are ranked by milligrams of vitamin E per standard amount. Adults need 15 milligrams per day (lactating women need 19 mg per day).

Food, Standard Amount	Vitamin E (mg)
Fortified ready-to-eat cereals, approximately 1 ounce	1.6–12.8
Sunflower seeds, dry roasted, 1 ounce	7.4
Almonds, 1 ounce	7.3
Sunflower oil, high linoleic, 1 tablespoon	5.6
Cottonseed oil, 1 tablespoon	4.8
Safflower oil, high oleic, 1 tablespoon	4.6
Hazelnuts (filberts), 1 ounce	4.3
Mixed nuts, dry roasted, 1 ounce	3.1
Turnip greens, frozen, cooked, ½ cup	2.9
Tomato paste, ¼ cup	2.8
Pine nuts, 1 ounce	2.6
Peanut butter, 2 tablespoons	2.5
Tomato puree, ½ cup	2.5
Tomato sauce, ½ cup	2.5
Canola oil, 1 tablespoon	2.4
Wheat germ, toasted, plain, 2 tablespoons	2.3
Peanuts, 1 ounce	2.2
Avocado, raw, ½ avocado	2.1
Carrot juice, canned, ¾ cup	2.1
Peanut oil, 1 tablespoon	2.1
Corn oil, 1 tablespoon	1.9
Olive oil, 1 tablespoon	1.9
Spinach, cooked, ½ cup	1.9
Dandelion greens, cooked, ½ cup	1.8
Sardine, Atlantic, in oil, drained, 3 ounces	1.7
Blue crab, cooked/canned, 3 ounces	1.6
Brazil nuts, 1 ounce	1.6
Herring, Atlantic, pickled, 3 ounces	1.5

Source: Nutrient values from the Agricultural Research Service (ARS) Nutrient Database for Standard Reference, Release 17. Foods are from the ARS single nutrient reports, sorted in descending order by nutrient content in terms of common household measures. Food items and weights in the single nutrient reports are adapted from those in the 2002 revision of USDA Home and Garden Bulletin no. 72, "Nutritive Value of Foods." Mixed dishes and multiple preparations of the same food item are omitted from this table.

Folate

Food sources are ranked by micrograms of folate per standard amount. All provide at least 10 percent of the RDA for folate for adults, which is 400 micrograms per day. Pregnant women (or those planning pregnancy) require 600 micrograms per day.

Food	Folate (µg)
Breakfast cereals[a] fortified with 100% of the daily value, ¾ cup	400
Beef liver, cooked, braised, 3 ounces	185
Cowpeas (black eyed), immature, cooked, boiled, ½ cup	105
Breakfast cereals[a] fortified with 25% of the daily value, ¾ cup	100
Spinach, frozen, cooked, boiled, ½ cup	100
Great Northern beans, boiled, ½ cup	90
Asparagus, boiled, 4 spears	85
Rice, white,[a] long grain, parboiled, enriched, cooked, ½ cup	65
Vegetarian baked beans, canned, 1 cup	60
Spinach, raw, 1 cup	60
Green peas, frozen, boiled, ½ cup	50
Broccoli, chopped, frozen, cooked, ½ cup	50
Egg noodles,[a] cooked, enriched, ½ cup	50
Broccoli, raw, 2 spears (each 5 inches long)	45
Avocado, raw, all varieties, sliced, ½ cup	45
Peanuts, all types, dry roasted, 1 ounce	40
Lettuce, romaine, shredded, ½ cup	40
Wheat germ, crude, 2 tablespoons	40
Tomato juice, canned, 6 ounces	35
Orange juice, chilled, includes concentrate, ¾ cup	35

[a]These items are fortified with folic acid as part of the Folate Fortification Program.

Source: U.S. Department of Agriculture, Agricultural Research Service, 2003. USDA National Nutrient Database for Standard Reference, Release 16. Nutrient Data Laboratory home page, www.nal.usda.gov/fnic/cgi-bin/nut_search.pl.

Vitamin B$_6$

Food sources are ranked by milligrams of vitamin B$_6$ per standard amount. Adults between the ages of nineteen and fifty need 1.3 milligrams per day. Pregnant and lactating women need between 1.9 and 2.0 milligrams per day, respectively. Women over fifty need 1.5 milligrams per day and men over fifty need 1.7 milligrams per day.

Food	Vitamin B$_6$ (mg)
Ready-to-eat cereal, 100% fortified, ¾ cup	2.00
Potato, baked, flesh and skin, 1 medium	0.70
Banana, raw, 1 medium	0.68
Garbanzo beans, canned, ½ cup	0.57
Chicken breast, meat only, cooked, ½ breast	0.52
Ready-to-eat cereal, 25% fortified, ¾ cup	0.50
Oatmeal, instant, fortified, 1 packet	0.42
Pork loin, lean only, cooked, 3 ounces	0.42
Roast beef, eye of round, lean only, cooked, 3 ounces	0.32
Trout, rainbow, cooked, 3 ounces	0.29
Sunflower seeds, kernels, dry roasted, 1 ounces	0.23
Spinach, frozen, cooked, ½ cup	0.14
Tomato juice, canned, 6 ounces	0.20
Avocado, raw, sliced, ½ cup	0.20
Salmon, sockeye, cooked, 3 ounces	0.19
Tuna, canned in water, drained solids, 3 ounces	0.18
Wheat bran, crude or unprocessed, ¼ cup	0.18
Peanut butter, smooth, 2 tablespoons	0.15
Walnuts, English/Persian, 1 ounce	0.15
Soybeans, green, boiled, drained, ½ cup	0.05
Lima beans, frozen, cooked, drained, ½ cup	0.10

Source: U.S. Department of Agriculture, Agricultural Research Service, 1999. USDA Nutrient Database for Standard Reference, Release 13. Nutrient Data Lab home page, www.nal.usda.gov/fnic/foodcomp.

Calcium: Dairy Sources

Food sources are ranked by milligrams of calcium per standard amount. Adults ages nineteen to fifty (including pregnant women) need 1,000 milligrams per day. Older adults need 1,200 milligrams per day.

Food, Standard Amount	Calcium (mg)
Plain yogurt, nonfat (13 g protein/8 ounces), 8-ounce container	452
Romano cheese, 1.5 ounces	452
Pasteurized process Swiss cheese, 2 ounces	438
Plain yogurt, low fat (12 g protein/8 ounces), 8-ounce container	415
Fruit yogurt, low fat (10 g protein/8 ounces), 8-ounce container	345
Swiss cheese, 1.5 ounces	336
Ricotta cheese, part skim, ½ cup	335
Pasteurized processed American cheese, 2 ounces	323
Provolone cheese, 1.5 ounces	321
Mozzarella cheese, part skim, 1.5 ounces	311
Cheddar cheese, 1.5 ounces	307
Fat-free (skim) milk, 1 cup	306
Muenster cheese, 1.5 ounces	305
1% low-fat milk, 1 cup	290
Low-fat chocolate milk (1%), 1 cup	288
2% reduced-fat milk, 1 cup	285
Reduced-fat chocolate milk (2%), 1 cup	285
Buttermilk, low fat, 1 cup	284
Chocolate milk, 1 cup	280
Whole milk, 1 cup	276
Yogurt, plain, whole milk (8 g protein/8 ounces), 8-ounce container	275
Ricotta cheese, whole milk, ½ cup	255
Blue cheese, 1.5 ounces	225
Mozzarella cheese, whole milk, 1.5 ounces	215
Feta cheese, 1.5 ounces	210

Source: Nutrient values from the Agricultural Research Service (ARS) Nutrient Database for Standard Reference, Release 17. Foods are from the ARS single nutrient reports, sorted in descending order by nutrient content in terms of common household measures. Food items and weights in the single nutrient reports are adapted from those in the 2002 revision of USDA Home and Garden Bulletin no. 72, "Nutritive Value of Foods." Mixed dishes and multiple preparations of the same food item are omitted from this table.

Calcium: Nondairy Sources

Food sources are ranked by milligrams of calcium per standard amount. Adults ages nineteen to fifty (including pregnant women) need 1,000 milligrams per day. Older adults need 1,200 milligrams per day. The bioavailability may vary.

Food, Standard Amount	Calcium (mg)[a]
Fortified ready-to-eat cereals (various), 1 ounce	236–1,043
Soy beverage, calcium fortified, 1 cup	368
Sardines, Atlantic, in oil, drained, 3 ounces	325
Tofu, firm, prepared with nigari,[b] ½ cup	253
Pink salmon, canned, with bone, 3 ounces	181
Collards, cooked from frozen, ½ cup	178
Molasses, blackstrap, 1 tablespoon	172
Spinach, cooked from frozen, ½ cup	146
Soybeans, green, cooked, ½ cup	130
Turnip greens, cooked from frozen, ½ cup	124
Ocean perch, Atlantic, cooked, 3 ounces	116
Oatmeal, plain and flavored, instant, fortified, 1 packet prepared	99–110
Cowpeas, cooked, ½ cup	106
White beans, canned, ½ cup	96
Kale, cooked from frozen, ½ cup	90
Okra, cooked from frozen, ½ cup	88
Soybeans, mature, cooked, ½ cup	88
Blue crab, canned, 3 ounces	86
Beet greens, cooked from fresh, ½ cup	82
Bok choy, Chinese cabbage, cooked from fresh, ½ cup	79
Clams, canned, 3 ounces	78
Dandelion greens, cooked from fresh, ½ cup	74
Rainbow trout, farmed, cooked, 3 ounces	73

[a] Both calcium content and bioavailability should be considered when selecting dietary sources of calcium. Some plant foods have calcium that is well absorbed, but the large quantity of plant foods that would be needed to provide as much calcium as in a glass of milk may be unachievable for many. Many other calcium-fortified foods are available, but the percentage of calcium that can be absorbed is unavailable for many of them.

[b] Calcium sulfate and magnesium chloride.

Source: Nutrient values from the Agricultural Research Service (ARS) Nutrient Database for Standard Reference, Release 17. Foods are from the ARS single nutrient reports, sorted in descending order by nutrient content in terms of common household measures. Food items and weights in the single nutrient reports are adapted from those in the 2002 revision of USDA Home and Garden Bulletin no. 72, "Nutritive Value of Foods." Mixed dishes and multiple preparations of the same food item are omitted from this table.

Potassium

Food sources ranked by milligrams of potassium per standard amount. Adults need 4,700 milligrams per day. Lactating women need 5,100 milligrams per day.

Food, Standard Amount	Potassium (mg)
Sweet potato, baked, 1 potato (146 g)	694
Tomato paste, ¼ cup	664
Beet greens, cooked, ½ cup	655
Potato, baked, flesh, 1 potato (156 g)	610
White beans, canned, ½ cup	595
Yogurt, plain, nonfat, 8-ounce container	579
Tomato purée, ½ cup	549
Clams, canned, 3 ounces	534
Yogurt, plain, low fat, 8-ounce container	531
Prune juice, ¾ cup	530
Carrot juice, ¾ cup	517
Blackstrap molasses, 1 tablespoon	498
Halibut, cooked, 3 ounces	490
Soybeans, green, cooked, ½ cup	485
Tuna, yellow fin, cooked, 3 ounces	484
Lima beans, cooked, ½ cup	484
Winter squash, cooked, ½ cup	448
Soybeans, mature, cooked, ½ cup	443
Rockfish, Pacific, cooked, 3 ounces	442
Cod, Pacific, cooked, 3 ounces	439
Bananas, 1 medium	422
Spinach, cooked, ½ cup	419
Tomato juice, ¾ cup	417
Tomato sauce, ½ cup	405
Peaches, dried, uncooked, ¼ cup	398
Prunes, stewed, ½ cup	398

Food, Standard Amount	Potassium (mg)
Milk, nonfat, 1 cup	382
Pork chop, center loin, cooked, 3 ounces	382
Apricots, dried, uncooked, ¼ cup	378
Rainbow trout, farmed, cooked, 3 ounces	375
Pork loin, center rib (roasts), lean, roasted, 3 ounces	371
Buttermilk, cultured, low fat, 1 cup	370
Cantaloupe, ¼ medium	368
1% or 2% milk, 1 cup	366
Honeydew melon, ⅛ medium	365
Lentils, cooked, ½ cup	365
Plantains, cooked, sliced, ½ cup	358
Kidney beans, cooked, ½ cup	358
Orange juice, ¾ cup	355
Split peas, cooked, ½ cup	355
Yogurt, plain, whole milk, 8-ounce container	352

Source: Nutrient values from the Agricultural Research Service (ARS) Nutrient Database for Standard Reference, Release 17. Foods are from the ARS single nutrient reports, sorted in descending order by nutrient content in terms of common household measures. Food items and weights in the single nutrient reports are adapted from those in the 2002 revision of USDA Home and Garden Bulletin no. 72, "Nutritive Value of Foods." Mixed dishes and multiple preparations of the same food item are omitted from this table.

Iron

Food sources are ranked by milligrams of iron per standard amount. Women between the ages of nineteen and fifty need 18 milligrams per day. Men and women older than fifty need 8 milligrams per day.

Food, Standard Amount	Iron (mg)
Clams, canned, drained, 3 ounces	23.8
Fortified ready-to-eat cereals (various), approximately 1 ounce	1.8–21.1
Oysters, eastern, wild, cooked, moist heat, 3 ounces	10.2
Organ meats (liver, giblets),[a] various, cooked, 3 ounces	5.2–9.9
Fortified instant cooked cereals (various), 1 packet	4.9–8.1
Soybeans, mature, cooked, ½ cup	4.4
Pumpkin and squash seed kernels, roasted, 1 ounce	4.2

Food, Standard Amount	Iron (mg)
White beans, canned, ½ cup	3.9
Blackstrap molasses, 1 tablespoon	3.5
Lentils, cooked, ½ cup	3.3
Spinach, cooked from fresh, ½ cup	3.2
Beef, chuck, blade roast, lean, cooked, 3 ounces	3.1
Beef, bottom round, lean, 0-inch fat, all grades, cooked, 3 ounces	2.8
Kidney beans, cooked, ½ cup	2.6
Sardines, canned in oil, drained, 3 ounces	2.5
Beef, rib, lean, ¼-inch fat, all grades, 3 ounces	2.4
Chickpeas, cooked, ½ cup	2.4
Duck, meat only, roasted, 3 ounces	2.3
Lamb, shoulder, arm, lean, ¼-inch fat, choice, cooked, 3 ounces	2.3
Prune juice, ¾ cup	2.3
Shrimp, canned, 3 ounces	2.3
Cowpeas, cooked, ½ cup	2.2
Ground beef, 15% fat, cooked, 3 ounces	2.2
Tomato purée, ½ cup	2.2
Lima beans, cooked, ½ cup	2.2
Soybeans, green, cooked, ½ cup	2.2
Navy beans, cooked, ½ cup	2.1
Refried beans, ½ cup	2.1
Beef, top sirloin, lean, 0-inch fat, all grades, cooked, 3 ounces	2.0
Tomato paste, ¼ cup	2.0

Source: Nutrient values from the Agricultural Research Service (ARS) Nutrient Database for Standard Reference, Release 17. Foods are from the ARS single nutrient reports, sorted in descending order by nutrient content in terms of common household measures. Food items and weights in the single nutrient reports are adapted from those in the 2002 revision of USDA Home and Garden Bulletin no. 72, "Nutritive Value of Foods." Mixed dishes and multiple preparations of the same food item are omitted from this table.

[a] High in cholesterol.

Magnesium

Food sources are ranked by milligrams of magnesium per standard amount. Women need between 310 and 320 milligrams per day and men need between 400 and 420 milligrams per day.

Food, Standard Amount	Magnesium (mg)
Pumpkin and squash seed kernels, roasted, 1 ounce	151
Brazil nuts, 1 ounce	107
Bran ready-to-eat cereal (100%), approximately 1 ounce	103
Halibut, cooked, 3 ounces	91
Quinoa, dry, ¼ cup	89
Spinach, canned, ½ cup	81
Almonds, 1 ounce	78
Spinach, cooked from fresh, ½ cup	78
Buckwheat flour, ¼ cup	75
Cashews, dry roasted, 1 ounce	74
Soybeans, mature, cooked, ½ cup	74
Pine nuts, dried, 1 ounce	71
Mixed nuts, oil roasted, with peanuts, 1 ounce	67
White beans, canned, ½ cup	67
Pollock, walleye, cooked, 3 ounces	62
Black beans, cooked, ½ cup	60
Bulgur, dry, ¼ cup	57
Oat bran, raw, ¼ cup	55
Soybeans, green, cooked, ½ cup	54
Tuna, yellowfin, cooked, 3 ounces	54
Artichokes (hearts), cooked, ½ cup	50
Peanuts, dry roasted, 1 ounce	50
Lima beans, baby, cooked from frozen, ½ cup	50
Beet greens, cooked, ½ cup	49
Navy beans, cooked, ½ cup	48
Tofu, firm, prepared with nigari[a], ½ cup	47
Okra, cooked from frozen, ½ cup	47
Soy beverage, 1 cup	47
Cowpeas, cooked, ½ cup	46
Hazelnuts, 1 ounce	46
Oat bran muffin, 1 ounce	45
Great Northern beans, cooked, ½ cup	44
Oat bran, cooked, ½ cup	44
Buckwheat groats, roasted, cooked, ½ cup	43

Food, Standard Amount	Magnesium (mg)
Brown rice, cooked, ½ cup	42
Haddock, cooked, 3 ounces	42

Source: Nutrient values from the Agricultural Research Service (ARS) Nutrient Database for Standard Reference, Release 17. Foods are from the ARS single nutrient reports, sorted in descending order by nutrient content in terms of common household measures. Food items and weights in the single nutrient reports are adapted from those in the 2002 revision of USDA Home and Garden Bulletin no. 72, "Nutritive Value of Foods." Mixed dishes and multiple preparations of the same food item are omitted from this table.

[a]Calcium sulfate and magnesium chloride.

Fiber

Food sources are ranked by grams of dietary fiber per standard amount. Women between the ages of nineteen and fifty need 25 grams per day; older women need 21 grams per day. Men between the ages of nineteen and fifty need 38 grams per day; older men need 30 grams per day.

Food, Standard Amount	Dietary Fiber (g)
Navy beans, cooked, ½ cup	9.5
Bran ready-to-eat cereal (100%), ½ cup	8.8
Kidney beans, canned, ½ cup	8.2
Split peas, cooked, ½ cup	8.1
Lentils, cooked, ½ cup	7.8
Black beans, cooked, ½ cup	7.5
Pinto beans, cooked, ½ cup	7.7
Lima beans, cooked, ½ cup	6.6
Artichoke, globe, cooked, 1 each	6.5
White beans, canned, ½ cup	6.3
Chickpeas, cooked, ½ cup	6.2
Great Northern beans, cooked, ½ cup	6.2
Cowpeas, cooked, ½ cup	5.6
Soybeans, mature, cooked, ½ cup	5.2
Bran ready-to-eat cereals, various, approximately 1 ounce	2.6–5.0
Crackers, rye wafers, plain, 2 wafers	5.0
Sweet potato, baked, with peel, 1 medium (146 g)	4.8
Asian pear, raw, 1 small	4.4
Green peas, cooked, ½ cup	4.4
Whole-wheat English muffin, 1 each	4.4

Food, Standard Amount	Dietary Fiber (g)
Pear, raw, 1 small	4.3
Bulgur, cooked, ½ cup	4.1
Mixed vegetables, cooked, ½ cup	4.0
Raspberries, raw, ½ cup	4.0
Sweet potato, boiled, no peel, 1 medium (156 g)	3.9
Blackberries, raw, ½ cup	3.8
Potato, baked, with skin, 1 medium	3.8
Soybeans, green, cooked, ½ cup	3.8
Stewed prunes, ½ cup	3.8
Figs, dried, ¼ cup	3.7
Dates, ¼ cup	3.6
Oat bran, raw, ¼ cup	3.6
Pumpkin, canned, ½ cup	3.6
Spinach, frozen, cooked, ½ cup	3.5
Shredded wheat ready-to-eat cereals, various, approximately 1 ounce	2.8–3.4
Almonds, 1 ounce	3.3
Apple with skin, raw, 1 medium	3.3
Brussels sprouts, frozen, cooked, ½ cup	3.2
Whole-wheat spaghetti, cooked, ½ cup	3.1
Banana, 1 medium	3.1
Orange, raw, 1 medium	3.1
Oat bran muffin, 1 small	3.0
Guava, 1 medium	3.0
Pearled barley, cooked, ½ cup	3.0
Sauerkraut, canned, solids, and liquids, ½ cup	3.0
Tomato paste, ¼ cup	2.9
Winter squash, cooked, ½ cup	2.9
Broccoli, cooked, ½ cup	2.8
Parsnips, cooked, chopped, ½ cup	2.8
Turnip greens, cooked, ½ cup	2.5
Collards, cooked, ½ cup	2.7
Okra, frozen, cooked, ½ cup	2.6
Peas, edible pods, cooked, ½ cup	2.5

Source: Nutrient Values from the Agricultural Research Service (ARS) Nutrient Database for Standard Reference, Release 17. Foods are from the ARS single nutrient reports, sorted in descending order by nutrient content in terms of common household measures. Food items and weights in the single nutrient reports are adapted from those in the 2002 revision of USDA Home and Garden Bulletin no. 72, "Nutritive Value of Foods." Mixed dishes and multiple preparations of the same food item are omitted.

APPENDIX E
What's a Portion?

The following chart will help you estimate portion sizes of many of the foods you consume, which is especially useful when you're on the run and can't measure how much you're having. Photocopy this list and keep it in your bag or wallet for quick reference.

Sizing Up Portion Sizes		
Food	**Amount**	**Looks Like**
Fresh fruit (like an apple or a peach)	1 (equals 1 cup fruit)	Tennis ball
Dried fruit	¼ cup (equals ½ cup fruit)	Golf ball
Berries	1 cup (equals 1 cup fruit)	Baseball
Baked potato or sweet potato	1 (equals 1 cup vegetable)	Computer mouse
Meat or poultry; fish such as tuna or salmon steak	1 ounce (equals a 1-ounce equivalent of meat/beans)	Matchbook
Meat or poultry; fish such as tuna or salmon steak	3 ounces (equals three 1-ounce equivalents of meat/beans)	Deck of cards
Fleshy white fish, such as flounder, sole, etc.	1 ounce (equals a 1-ounce equivalent of meat/beans)	Matchbook
Fleshy white fish, such as flounder, sole, etc.	3 ounces (equals three 1-ounce equivalent of meat/beans)	Checkbook
Peanut butter	2 tablespoons (equals two 1-ounce equivalent of meat/beans plus 2 oils)	Walnut in the shell
Nuts	1 ounce (equals two 1-ounce equivalents of meat/beans plus 2 oils)	1 small handful
Hard cheese	1½ ounces (equals 1 milk/yogurt/cheese)	6 dice
Ready-to-eat cereal, rice, or pasta	1 cup (equals 1 grain)	Baseball
Popcorn	3 cups (equals 1 grain)	3 baseballs

Food	Amount	Looks Like
Pancake or waffle (4-inch diameter)	1 (equals 1 grain)	Diameter of a compact disc
Salad dressing	2 tablespoons (equals 2 oils)	Shot glass
Oil (e.g., olive, canola, etc.)	1 teaspoon (equals 1 oil)	Standard cap of a 16-ounce water bottle
Margarine or mayonnaise	1 teaspoon (equals 1 oil)	Standard postal stamp

Adapted with permission from L. R. Young, The Portion Teller, *New York: Morgan Road Books, 2005.*

APPENDIX F
All about Exercise

How many calories does physical activity use? A 154-pound, five foot ten man will use up about the number of calories listed in the following table doing each activity listed. Men and women who weigh more will use more calories, and those who weigh less, including children, will use fewer.

Approximate Calories Used by a 154-Pound Man		
	In 1 Hour	In 30 Minutes
Moderate Physical Activities:		
Hiking	370	185
Light gardening/yard work	330	165
Dancing	330	165
Golf (walking and carrying clubs)	330	165
Bicycling (less than 10 miles per hour)	290	145
Walking (3½ miles per hour)	280	140
Weight training (general light workout)	220	110
Stretching	180	90
Vigorous Physical Activities:		
Running/jogging (5 miles per hour)	590	295
Bicycling (more than 10 miles per hour)	590	295
Swimming (slow freestyle laps)	510	255
Aerobics	480	240
Walking (4½ miles per hour)	460	230
Heavy yard work (chopping wood)	440	220
Weight lifting (vigorous effort)	440	220
Basketball (vigorous)	440	220

Exercise During Pregnancy

According to the American College of Obstetricians and Gynecologists (ACOG) guidelines released in 2002 (committee opinion no. 267: "Exercise during Pregnancy and the Postpartum Period," 99:171–73), unless there are medical reasons to avoid it, pregnant women can do about 30 minutes of moderate exercise on most, if not all, days. Women should check with a health-care provider before doing any exercise while pregnant. Brisk walking, dancing, swimming, biking, aerobics, or yoga are safe options, but pregnant women should avoid activities that present a high risk for injury, such as horseback riding or downhill skiing. They should also avoid sports in which they could get hit in the abdomen, especially after the third month, or in their backs. Scuba diving should be avoided because it can cause dangerous gas bubbles in the baby's circulatory system.

APPENDIX G
Master Food Lists

The following tables contain a list for each of the food categories recommended in chapter 10. Use these tables to find approximate measures of many of the foods and beverages you and your family consume.

Fruit		
Type of Fruit	**½ Cup of Fruit Equals**	**1 Cup of Fruit Equals**
Apple	½ cup sliced or chopped, raw or cooked	½ large (3¼-inch diameter) 1 small (2½-inch diameter) 1 cup sliced or chopped, raw or cooked
Applesauce	1 snack container (4 ounces)	1 cup
Banana	1 small (less than 6 inches long)	1 cup sliced 1 large (8 to 9 inches long)
Cantaloupe	1 medium wedge (⅛ medium melon)	1 cup diced or melon balls
Grapes	16 seedless grapes	1 cup whole or cut-up 32 seedless grapes
Grapefruit	½ medium (4-inch diameter)	1 medium (4-inch diameter) 1 cup sections
Mixed fruit (fruit cocktail)	1 snack container (4 ounces) drained (⅜ cup)	1 cup diced or sliced, raw or canned, drained
Orange	1 small (2⅜-inch diameter)	1 large (3 1/16-inch diameter) 1 cup sections
Orange, mandarin	½ cup canned, drained	1 cup canned, drained
Peach	1 small (2⅜-inch diameter) 1 snack container (4 ounces) drained = ⅜ cup	1 large (2¾-inch diameter) 1 cup sliced or diced, raw, cooked, or canned, drained 2 halves, canned

Fruit (*continued*)

Type of Fruit	½ Cup of Fruit Equals	1 Cup of Fruit Equals
Pear	1 snack container (4 ounces) drained = ⅜ cup ½ cup sliced or diced, raw, cooked, or canned, drained	1 medium pear (2½ per pound) 1 cup sliced or diced, raw, cooked, or canned, drained
Pineapple	1 snack container (4 ounces) drained = ⅜ cup ½ cup chunks, sliced or crushed, raw, cooked, or canned, drained	1 cup chunks, sliced or crushed, raw, cooked, or canned, drained
Plum	1 large plum	1 cup sliced raw or cooked 3 medium or 2 large plums
Strawberries	½ cup whole, haved, or sliced, fresh or frozen	About 8 large berries 1 cup whole, halved, or sliced, fresh or frozen
Watermelon	6 melon balls	1 small wedge (1-inch thick) 1 cup diced or balls
Dried fruit (raisins, prunes, apricots, etc.)	¼ cup dried fruit = ½ cup fruit (1 small box of raisins, 1½ ounces)	½ cup dried fruit = 1 cup fruit
100% fruit juice (orange, apple, grape, grapefruit, etc.)	½ cup (4 ounces)	1 cup (8 ounces)

Vegetables

Type of Vegetable	½ Cup of Vegetables Equals	1 Cup of Vegetables Equals
Broccoli	½ cup chopped or florets 1½ spears 5-inches long raw or cooked	1 cup chopped or florets 3 spears 5-inches long raw or cooked
Greens (collards, mustard greens, turnip greens, kale)	½ cup cooked	1 cup cooked
Spinach	1 cup raw = ½ cup vegetables	1 cup cooked or 2 cups raw = 1 cup vegetables
Raw leafy greens: spinach, romaine, watercress, dark green leafy lettuce, endive, escarole	1 cup raw = ½ cup vegetables	2 cups raw = 1 cup vegetables
Carrots	½ cup strips, slices, or chopped, raw or cooked	1 cup strips, or chopped, raw or cooked
6 baby carrots	1 medium carrot	2 medium carrots 1 cup baby carrots (12)

Type of Vegetable	½ Cup of Vegetables Equals	1 Cup of Vegetables Equals
Pumpkin	½ cup mashed, cooked	1 cup mashed, cooked
Sweet potatoes	½ large baked (2½-inch or more diameter) ½ cup sliced, mashed, or cooked	1 large baked (2½-inch or more diameter) 1 cup sliced, mashed, or cooked
Winter squash (acorn, butternut, or hubbard)	½ acorn squash, baked = ¾ cup	1 cup cubed, cooked
Dry beans and peas (such as black, garbanzo, kidney, pinto, or soy beans, or black eyed peas or split peas)	½ cup whole or mashed, cooked	1 cup whole or mashed, cooked
Tofu	1 piece 2½ x 2¾ by 1-inch (about 4 ounces)	1 cup ½-inch cubes (about 8 ounces)
Corn, yellow and white	½ cup 1 small ear (about 6 inches long)	1 cup 1 large ear (8 to 9 inches long)
Green peas	½ cup	1 cup
White potatoes	½ cup diced, mashed ½ medium boiled or baked potato (2½- to 3-inch diameter)	1 cup diced, mashed 1 medium boiled or baked potato (2½- to 3- inch diameter)
Bean sprouts	½ cup cooked	1 cup cooked
Cabbage, green	½ cup chopped, shredded, raw or cooked	1 cup chopped, shredded, raw or cooked
Cauliflower	½ cup pieces or florets raw or cooked	1 cup pieces or florets raw or cooked
Celery	½ cup diced or sliced, raw or cooked 1 large stalk (11 to 12 inches long)	1 cup diced or sliced, raw or cooked 2 large stalks (11 to 12 inches long)
Cucumbers	½ cup raw, sliced or chopped	1 cup raw, sliced or chopped
Green or wax beans	½ cup cooked	1 cup cooked
Green or red peppers	½ cup chopped, raw or cooked 1 small pepper	1 cup chopped, raw or cooked 1 large pepper (3-inch diameter, 3¾ inches long)
Lettuce, iceberg or head	1 cup raw, shredded or chopped	2 cups raw, shredded or chopped
Mushrooms	½ cup raw or cooked	1 cup raw or cooked
Onions	½ cup chopped, raw or cooked	1 cup chopped, raw or cooked
Tomatoes	1 small raw whole (2¼ inches) 1 medium canned	1 large raw whole (3 inches) 1 cup chopped or sliced, raw, canned, or cooked

Vegetables (*continued*)

Type of Vegetable	½ Cup of Vegetables Equals	1 Cup of Vegetables Equals
Tomato or mixed vegetable juice	½ cup	1 cup
Summer squash or zucchini	½ cup cooked, sliced or diced	1 cup cooked, sliced or diced

Grains

Type of Grain	A 1-Ounce Equivalent Equals
Bagels	½ "mini" bagel
Breads (whole wheat, whole grain, white)	1 regular slice 1 small slice French 4 snack-size
Bulgur (cracked wheat)	½ cup cooked
Crackers (100% whole wheat, rye, saltines, snack crackers)	5 whole wheat crackers 2 rye crisp breads 7 square or round crackers
English muffins (whole wheat, whole grain)	½ muffin
Muffin (bran, oat)	½ medium (about 1 ounce)
Oatmeal	½ cup cooked 1 packet instant 1 ounce dry (regular or quick)
Pancakes (whole wheat, buckwheat, buttermilk, plain)	1 pancake (4 ½-inch diameter) 2 small pancakes (3-inch diameter)
Popcorn (air-popped)	3 cups, popped
Ready-to-eat breakfast cereal (whole wheat, whole oat, bran, whole grain)	1 cup flakes or rounds 1¼ cup puffed
Rice (brown, wild, white)	½ cup cooked 1 ounce dry
Pasta—spaghetti, macaroni, noodles (whole wheat)	½ cup cooked 1 ounce dry
Tortillas (whole wheat, white, corn)	1 small flour tortilla (6-inch diameter) 1 corn tortilla (6-inch diameter)

Milk

Type of Milk	A 1-Cup Equivalent Equals
Skim milk	1 cup 1 half-pint container ½ cup evaporated milk
Yogurt (low fat or nonfat, plain)	1 regular container (8 fluid ounces) 1 cup

Type of Milk	A 1-Cup Equivalent Equals
Cheese (low fat or fat free)	1½ ounces hard cheese (cheddar, mozzarella, Swiss, parmesan) ⅓ cup shredded cheese 2 ounces processed cheese (American) ½ cup ricotta cheese 2 cups cottage cheese
Milk-based desserts (fat free or low fat)	1 cup pudding made with milk 1 cup frozen yogurt

Meat and Beans

Type of Meat or Bean	Amount that Counts as a 1-Ounce Equivalent
Meats	1 ounce cooked lean beef 1 ounce cooked lean pork or ham
Poultry	1 ounce cooked chicken or turkey, without skin 1 sandwich slice of turkey (4½ by 2½ by ⅛ inch)
Fish	1 ounce cooked fish or shellfish
Eggs	1 egg 3 egg whites
Nuts and seeds	½ ounce of nuts (12 almonds, 24 pistachios, 7 walnut halves) ½ ounce of seeds (pumpkin, sunflower or squash seeds, hulled, roasted) 1 Tablespoon of peanut butter or almond butter
Dry beans and peas	¼ cup of cooked dry beans (such as black, kidney, pinto, or white beans) ¼ cup of cooked dry peas (such as chickpeas, cowpeas, lentils, or split peas) ¼ cup of baked beans, refried beans ¼ cup (about 2 ounces) of tofu 1 ounce tempeh, cooked ¼ cup roasted soybeans 1 falafel patty (2¼ inches, 4 ounces) 2 tablespoons hummus

Extra Calories

Food or Beverage	Counts As
Beef bologna, 3 1-ounce slices	3 meat and beans plus 100 extra calories
Beef sausage, pre-cooked, 3 ounces	3 meat and beans plus 180 extra calories
Biscuit, plain, 1-2½-inch diameter	1 grain plus 60 extra calories
Blueberry muffin, 1 small (2 ounces)	1½ grain plus 45 extra calories

Extra Calories (*continued*)

Food or Beverage	Counts As
Butter, 1 teaspoon	35 extra calories
Cheese sauce, ¼ cup	1 milk plus 75 extra calories
Cheese, whole milk mozzarella, 1½ ounces	1 milk plus 45 extra calories
Cinnamon sweet roll, 1 3-ounce roll	2 grains plus 100 extra calories
Coconut oil or palm kernel oil, 1 tablespoon	120 extra calories
Cornbread, 1 piece (2½ by 2½ by 1¾ inches)	1½ grain plus 50 extra calories
Cream cheese, 1 tablespoon	50 extra calories
Croissant, 1 medium, 2 ounces	1½ grain plus 95 extra calories
French fries, 1 medium order	1 cup vegetables plus 325 extra calories
Fried chicken with skin and batter, 3 wings	3 meat and beans plus 335 extra calories
Frozen yogurt, 1 cup	1 milk plus 140 extra calories
Fruit punch, 1 cup (8 fluid ounces)	115 extra calories
Glazed doughnut, yeast type, 1 medium, 3¾-inch diameter	1 grain plus 50 extra calories
Half and half, 1 tablespoon	20 extra calories
Heavy (whipping) cream, 1 tablespoon	50 extra calories
Ice cream, vanilla, 1 cup	1 milk plus 205 extra calories
Onion rings, 1 order (8 to 9 rings)	1 cup vegetables plus 160 extra calories
Pork sausage, 3 ounces cooked	3 meat and beans plus 125 extra calories
Regular ground beef, 80% lean, 3 ounces	3 meat and beans plus 65 extra calories
Roasted chicken thigh with skin, 3 ounces	3 meat and beans plus 70 extra calories
Soda, 1 bottle (20 fluid ounces)	260 extra calories
Soda, 1 can (12 fluid ounces)	155 extra calories
Stick margarine, 1 teaspoon	35 extra calories

Resources

Healthy Eating and Weight Management

America on the Move
Sponsored by the not-for-profit Partnership to Promote Healthy Eating and
Active Living, America on the Move is a national program that supports
small changes in eating and lifestyle habits in our society.
www.americaonthemove.org

Centers for Disease Control and Prevention
www.cdc.gov

Dietary Guidelines for Americans 2005, Sixth Edition
United States Department of Health and Human Services (HHS) and the
United States Department of Agriculture (USDA)
www.healthierus.gov/dietaryguidelines

Dietary Guidelines for Americans Advisory Committee Report, 2005
www.health.gov/dietaryguidelines/dga2005/report

Dietary Reference Intakes
These comprehensive tables from the National Academy of Sciences Institute of Medicine, Food and Nutrition Board list recommended intakes of
vitamins, minerals, and macronutrients. They are organized by age and
gender.
www.iom.edu/Object.File/Master/21/372/0.pdf

Food Allergy and Anaphylaxis Network
The Food Allergy and Anaphylaxis Network (FAAN), established in 1991,
raises awareness of food allergy and anaphylaxis, provides advocacy and

education, and supports and conducts research on food allergies and anaphylaxis.
11781 Lee Jackson Highway, Suite 160
Fairfax, VA 22033-3309
1-800-929-4040
www.foodallergy.org

Food Safety
The following Web sites provide information for food safety including safe
food-storage tips:
www.foodsafety.gov/
www.homefoodsafety.org
www.fda.gov/womens/healthinformation/pregnancy.html

Media-Smart Youth: Eat, Think, and Be Active!
This is an after-school program that targets students between ages eleven
and thirteen and helps them become aware of how the media influences
their food choices.
1-800-370-2943
www.nichd.nih.gov/msy

MyPyramid, the New Food Guidance System (USDA)
www.mypyramid.gov

National Diabetes Information Clearinghouse
1 Information Way
Bethesda, MD 20892-3560
301-654-3327
www.fda.gov/diabetes

National Heart, Lung, and Blood Institute
P.O. Box 30105
Bethesda, MD 20824-0105
301-251-1222
www.nhlbi.nih.gov

National Institute of Diabetes and Digestive and Kidney Diseases
31 Center Drive, MSC-2560
Building 31, Room 9A-04
Bethesda, MD 20892-2560
301-496-3583
www.niddk.nih.gov

National Sleep Foundation
1522 K Street, NW, Suite 500
Washington, DC 20005
202-347-3471
www.sleepfoundation.org

United States Department of Health and Human Services (HHS)
200 Independence Avenue, SW
Washington, DC 20201
202-619-0257
1-877-696-6775
www.hhs.gov

www.healthierus.gov
This Web site from HHS provides great information on nutrition and physical fitness and provides links to a variety of government-sponsored health Web sites.

United States Department of Agriculture Center for Nutrition Policy and Promotion
3101 Park Center Drive, Room 1034
Alexandria, VA 22302-1594
www.usda.gov/cnpp

www.nal.usda.gov/fnic/foodcomp
This Web site from the USDA provides food composition data (for example, calories) for more than 7,300 foods available in the United States.

www.nal.usda.gov/fnic/etext/000106.html
This Food and Nutrition Information Center from the USDA has a lot of information about pregnancy, breast-feeding, infant and child nutrition, as well as other topics that relate to feeding yourself and your family.

United States Food and Drug Administration (FDA)
5600 Fishers Lane
Rockville, MD 20857-0001
1-888-INFO-FDA (1-888-463-6332)
www. FDA.gov
For information about the Nutrition Facts Panels on food products, see www.cfsan.fda.gov/~dms/foodlab.html.
For information about Qualified Health Claims on food product labels, see www.cfsan.fda.gov/~dms/lab-qhc.html.

We Can
We Can! Ways to Enhance Children's Activity & Nutrition, created by HHS and NIH, is a national education program designed for parents and caregivers to help children eight to thirteen years old stay at a healthy weight.
www.nhlbi.nih.gov/health/public/heart/obesity/wecan/

Weight Control Information Network
The Weight Control Information Network, created by HHS and NIH, provides information on weight control, obesity, physical activity, and related nutritional issues.
1-800-WIN-8098
www.win.niddk.nih.gov/index.htm

Professional Organizations

Allergy and Asthma Network: Mothers of Asthmatics
2751 Prosperity Avenue, Suite 150
Fairfax, VA 22031
800-878-4403
www.aanma.org

American Academy of Allergy, Asthma and Immunology (AAAAI)
611 East Wells Street
Milwaukee, WI 53202
AAAAI Physician Referral and Information Line: 800-822-2762
www.aaaai.org

American Cancer Society
Atlanta, Georgia
1-800-ACS-2345
www.cancer.org

American College of Obstetrics and Gynecology
www.acog.org

American College of Sports Medicine
P.O. Box 1440
Indianapolis, IN 46206-1440
317-637-9200
Fax: 317-634-7817
www.acsm.org

American Diabetes Association
National Call Center
1701 North Beauregard Street
Alexandria, VA 22311
1-800-DIABETES
1-800-342-2383
Fax: 815-734-1223
www.diabetes.org
askADA@diabetes.org

American Dietetic Association
120 S. Riverside Plaza, Suite 2000
Chicago, IL 60606-6995
800-877-1600
Fax: 312-899-1979
www.eatright.org
To find a registered dietitian in your area, call 1-800-366-1655.

American Obesity Association
1250 24th Street, NW, Suite 300
Washington, DC 20037
800-98-OBESE
www.obesity.org

Center for Science in the Public Interest (CSPI)
1875 Connecticut Avenue, NW, Suite 300
Washington, DC 20009-5728
202-332-9110
Fax: 202-265-4954
www.cspinet.org

National Cancer Institute
Office of Cancer Communications
9000 Rockville Pike
Building 31, Room 10A-24
Bethesda, MD 20892
800-4-CANCER (800-422-6237)
www.nci.nih.gov

North American Association for the Study of Obesity (NAASO)
8630 Fenton Street, Suite 918
Silver Spring, MD 20910
301-563-6526
Fax: 301-587-6595
www.naaso.org

National Eating Disorders Association
603 Stewart Street, Suite 803
Seattle, WA 98101
Business Office: 206-382-3587
Toll free Information and Referral Helpline 800-931-2237
info@NationalEatingDisorders.org

Shape Up America!
This nonprofit organization provides information to promote healthy
weight management in children.
www.shapeup.org

Other Resources

Environmental Nutrition: The Newsletter of Food, Nutrition and Health
P.O. Box 5656
Norwalk, CT 06856-5656
Customer_Service@belvoir.com
1-800-424-7887
www.environmentalnutrition.com

Nutrition Action Healthletter
Published by CSPI
www.cspinet.org/nah/index.htm
circ@cspinet.org

Tufts Health and Nutrition Letter
www.healthletter.tufts.edu

Selected References

American Heart Association, S. S. Gidding, B. A. Dennison, L. L. Birch, S. R. Daniels, M. W. Gilman, A. H. Lichtenstein, K. T. Rattay, J. Steinberger, N. Stettler, and L. Van Horn. 2006. Dietary recommendations for children and adolescents: a guide for practitioners. *Pediatrics* 117(2):544–559.

Berkowitz, R. I., V. A. Stallings, G. Maislin, and A. J. Stunkard. 2005. Growth of children at high risk of obesity during the first 6 y of life: implications for prevention. *American Journal of Clinical Nutrition* 81(1):140–146.

Bowman, S. A., S. L. Gortmaker, C. B. Ebbeling, M. A. Pereira, and D. S. Ludwig. 2004. Effects of fast-food consumption on energy intake and diet quality among children in a national household survey. *Pediatrics* 113(1):112–118.

Brown, J. E. and M. Carlson. 2000. Nutrition and multifetal pregnancy. *Journal of the American Dietetic Association* 100:343–348.

Centers for Disease Control and Prevention. 2006. Youth Risk Behavior Surveillance—United States, 2005. *Morbidity & Mortality Weekly Report 55* (SS-5): 1–108.

Cordain, L., B. A. Watkins, G. L. Florant, M. Kelher, L. Rogers, and Y. Li. 2002. Fatty acid analysis of wild ruminant tissues: evolutionary implications for reducing diet-related chronic disease. *European Journal of Clinical Nutrition* 56(3):181–91.

Daniels, S.R., T. R. Kimball, J. A. Morrison, P. Khoury, S. Witt, and R. A. Meyer. 1995. Effect of lean body mass, fat mass, blood pressure, and sexual maturation on left ventricular mass in children and adolescents: statistical, biological and clinical significance. *Circulation* 92:3249–54.

de Souza, P., and K. E. Ciclitira. 2005. Men and dieting: a qualitative analysis. *Journal of Health Psychology* 10:793–804.

Ebbeling, C. B., K. B. Sinclair, M. A. Pereira, E. Garcia-Lago, H. A. Feldman, and D.S. Ludwig, 2004. Compensation for energy intake from fast food among overweight and lean adolescents. *Journal of the American Medical Association* 291(23):2828–33.

Fabricatore, A. N. and T. A. Wadden. 2006. *Annual Review of Clinical Psychology* 2:357–77.

Farrow, C., and J. Blissett. 2006. Does maternal control during feeding moderate early infant weight gain? *Pediatrics* 118(2):e293–98.

Fiocci, A., A. Assa'ad, and S. Bahna. 2006. Food allergy and the introduction of solid foods to infants: a consensus document. *Annals of Allergy, Asthma, and Immunology* 97(1):10–21.

Food and Nutrition Board, Institute of Medicine. 1990. *Nutrition during pregnancy*. Washington, DC: National Academy Press.

Forshee, R. A., P. A. Anderson, and M. L. Storey. 2006. Changes in calcium intake and association with beverage consumption and demographics: comparing data from CSFII 1994–1996, 1998 and NHANES 1999–2002. *Journal of the American College of Nutrition* 25(2):108–16.

Friedman, J. 2006. Molecular studies of food intake and body weight. *Howard Hughes Medical Institute Bulletin*. January 13, 2006.

Gangwisch, J. E., D. Malaspina, B. Boden-Albala, and S. B. Heymsfield. 2005. Inadequate sleep as a risk factor for obesity: analyses of the NHANES I. *Sleep* 28(10):1289–96.

Goodpaster, B. H., S. Krishnaswami, T. B. Harris, A. Katsiaras, S. B. Kritchevsky, E. M. Simonsick, M. Nevitt, P. Holvoet, and A. B. Newman. 2005. Obesity, regional body fat distribution, and the metabolic syndrome in older men and women. *Archives of Internal Medicine* 165:777–83.

Hanson, N. I., D. Neumark-Stainer, M. E. Eisenberg, M. Story, and M. Wall. 2005. Associations between parental report of the home food environment and adolescent intakes of fruits, vegetables and dairy foods. *Public Health Nutrition* 8(1):77–85.

Jakicic, J. M., R. R. Wing, B. A. Butler, and R. J. Robertson. 1995. *International Journal of Obesity and Related Metabolic Disorders* 19(12):893–901.

Judex, S., R. Garman, M. Squire, L. Donahue, and C. Rubin. 2004. Genetically based influences on the site-specific regulation of trabecular and cortical bone morphology. *Journal of Bone and Mineral Research* 19:600–6.

Lethbridge-Cejku, M., D. Rose, and J. Vickerie. 2006. Summary health statistics for U.S. adults: national health interview survey, 2004. National Center for Health Statistics. Vital Health Statistics. 10(2):18–19.

Lovejoy, J. C. 2003. The menopause and obesity. *Primary Care* 30(2):317–25.

Neumark-Sztainer, D., M. Wall, J. Guo, M. Story, J. Haines, and M. Eisenberg. 2006. Obesity, disordered eating, and eating disorders in a longitudinal study of adolescents: how do dieters fare 5 years later? *Journal of the American Dietetic Association* 106(4), 559–67.

Ogden, C.L., M. D. Carroll, L. R. Curtin, M. A. McDowell, C. J. Tabak, and K. M. Flegal. 2006. Prevalence of overweight and obesity in the United States, 1999–2004. *Journal of the American Medical Association* 295:1549–55.

Patton, G. C., R. Selzer, C. Coffey, J. B. Carlin, and R. Wolfe. 1999. Onset of adolescent eating disorders: population based cohort study over 3 years. *British Medical Journal* 318:765–68.

Phillips, S. M., L. G. Bandini, E. N. Naumova, H. Cyr, S. Colclough, W. H. Dietz, and A. Must. 2004. Energy-dense snack food intake in adolescence: longitudinal relationships to weight and fatness. *Obesity Research* 12:461–72.

Ritchie, L. D., P. B. Crawford, D. M. Hoelscher, and M. S. Sothern. 2006. Position of the American Dietetic Association: individual-, family-, school-, and community-based interventions for pediatric overweight. *Journal of the American Dietetic Association* 106(6):925–51.

Stice, E., K. Presnell, H. Shaw, and P. Rohde. 2005. Psychological and behavioral risk factors for obesity onset in adolescent girls. *Journal of Consulting and Clinical Psychology* 73(2):195–202.

Sternfeld, B., A. K. Bhat, H. Wang, T. Sharp, and C. P. Quesenberry, Jr. 2005. Menopause, physical activity, and body composition/fat distribution in midlife women. *Medicine and Science in Sports and Exercise* 37(7):1195–1202.

Sternfeld, B., H. Wang, C. P. Quesenberry Jr., B. Abrams, S. A. Everson-Rose, G. A. Greendale, K. A. Matthews, J. I. Torrens, and M. Sowers. 2004. Physical Activity and changes in weight and waist circumference in midlife women: findings from the Study of Women's Health Across the Nation. *American Journal of Epidemiology* 160(9):912–22.

Taylor, C. B., S. Bryson, A. A. Celio Doyle, K. H. Luce, D. Cunning, L. B. Abascal, R. Rockwell, A. E. Field, R. Striegel-Moore, A. J. Winzelberg, and D. E. Wilfey. 2006. The adverse effect of negative comments about weight and shape from family and siblings on women at high risk for eating disorders. *Pediatrics* 118(2):731–38.

U.S. Department of Health and Human Services. 2004. *Bone Health and Osteoporosis: A Report of the Surgeon General.* Rockville, MD: U.S. Department of Health and Human Services, Office of the Surgeon General.

Wahrenberg, H., K. Hertel, B. M. Leijonhufvud, L. G. Persson, E. Toft, and P. Arner. 2005. Use of waist circumference to predict insulin resistance: retrospective study. *British Medical Journal* 330:1,363–64.

Winter, R. 2004. *A Consumer's Dictionary of Food Additives: Descriptions in Plain English of More Than 12,000 Ingredients Both Harmful and Desirable Found in Foods*, 6th ed. New York, NY: Three Rivers Press.

Wright, J. D., J. Kennedy-Stephenson, C. Y. Wang, M. A. McDowell, C. L. Johnson, and the National Center for Health Statistics, CDC. 2004. Trends in intake of energy and macronutrients, United States, 1971–2000. *Morbidity and Mortality Weekly Report* 53(04):80–82.

Zied, E., and R. Winter. 2006. *So What Can I Eat?!* Hoboken, NJ: John Wiley and Sons, Inc.

Index